Authorised by the

Practical
First Aid

British Red Cross Chief Medical Advisor
Dr Vivien J Armstrong FRCA DRCOG PGCE (FE)

LONDON, NEW YORK,
MUNICH, MELBOURNE, AND DELHI

DORLING KINDERSLEY
Senior Art Editor Glenda Fisher
DTP Designer Sonia Charbonnier
Production Controller Elizabeth Cherry
Jacket designer Neal Cobourne
Managing Editor Penny Warren
Managing Art Editor Marianne Markham

Produced for Dorling Kindersley by
COOLING BROWN

Creative Director Arthur Brown
Project Editor Jemima Dunne
Designers Tish Jones, Peter Cooling

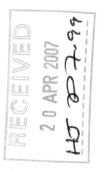

The material in this book reflects current first-aid practice at the time of publication but cannot be a substitute for actual training. For information on training programmes contact your local British Red Cross office.

For convenience and clarity, we have used the pronoun "he" when referring to the first aider or casualty, unless the individual in the accompanying photograph is female.

First published in the United Kingdom in 2003

This revised edition published in 2006 by
Dorling Kindersley Limited,
80 Strand, London WC2R 0RL

A Penguin Company

2 4 6 8 10 9 7 5 3 1

A CIP catalogue record for this book is available from the British Library.

ISBN 10: 1-4053-1952-6
ISBN 13: 978-1-4053-1952-2

Reproduced in Singapore by Colourscan
Printed and bound in China by WKT

Discover more at
www.dk.com

Contents

How to use this book 6

1 First-aid principles 7

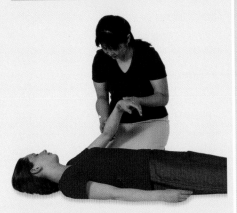

Dealing with an incident 8
Assessing dangers 10
Avoiding cross-infection 13
Managing an incident 14
Coping with stress 15
Initial assessment of a casualty 16
Detailed assessment of a casualty . . . 17
Carrying out a head-to-toe survey . . 18
Monitoring vital signs 20
First-aid materials 22
Sterile wound dressings 24
Plasters 25
Cold compresses 25
Roller bandages 26
Triangular bandages 27
Arm sling 28
Elevation sling 29
Test yourself 30

2 Life-saving techniques 31

Dealing with unconsciousness 32
Breathing and blood circulation 34
How resuscitation works 35
Resuscitation techniques 36
Check response (adult) 37
Check breathing (adult) 37
Recovery position (adult) 38
Chest compressions (adult) 40
Rescue breathing (adult) 42
Using a defibrillator 44
Check response (child) 46
Check breathing (child) 46
Recovery position (child) 47
Rescue breathing (child) 48
Chest compressions (child) 49
Check response (infant) 50
Check breathing (infant) 50
Recovery position (infant) 51
Rescue breathing (infant) 51
Chest compressions (infant) 52
Choking (adult) 53
Choking (child) 54
Choking (infant) 55
Test yourself 56

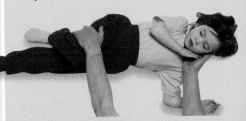

3 Wounds and bleeding   57

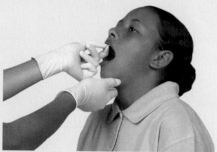

Dealing with severe bleeding 58
Blood vessels and bleeding 60
Shock 61
Cuts and grazes 62
Bruising 63
Blisters 63
Crush injury 64
Amputation 65
Eye wound 66
Scalp wound 66
Nosebleed 67
Ear wound 67
Mouth wound 68
Knocked-out tooth 68
Wound to palm 69
Embedded object 70
Splinters 72
Fish-hook injury 73
Test yourself 74

4 Environmental injuries   75

Dealing with severe burns 76
Types of burn 78
Minor burns and scalds 79
Face and head burns 80
Chemical burns 81
Electrical burns 82
Sunburn 83
Dehydration 84
Heat exhaustion 84
Heatstroke 85
Hypothermia 86
Frostbite 87
Test yourself 88

5 Disorders affecting consciousness   89

Dealing with a collapsed person 90
The nervous system 92
Head injury 93
Concussion 94
Compression 95
Stroke 96
Fainting 97
Epilepsy 98
Seizures in children . . . 99
Test yourself 100

6 Bone, joint, and muscle injuries 101

Dealing with a broken bone 102
Types of bone, joint,
    and muscle injury 104
Jaw injury 106
Cheek and nose injury 106
Collarbone injury 107
Arm injury 108
Hand and finger injury 108
Rib injury 109
Pelvic injury 109
Spinal injury 110
Leg injury 111
Ankle injury 112
Knee injury 113
Cramp 113
Test yourself 114

7 Poisoning, bites, and stings 115

Dealing with poisoning 116
Alcohol and drug poisoning 118
Insect stings 119
Snake bites 120
Animal bites 121
Marine injuries . . . 121
Test yourself 122

8 Medical problems and emergencies 123

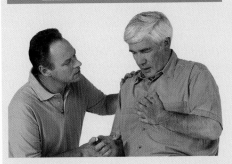

Dealing with a heart attack 124
Angina 126
Diabetic emergency 127
Allergy 128
Anaphylactic shock 129
Asthma 130
Croup 131
Object in the eye 132
Object in the ear 133
Object in the nose 133
Toothache 134
Earache 134
Headache 135
Migraine 135
Sore throat 136
Fever 136
Meningitis 137
Abdominal pain 138
Vomiting and diarrhoea 138
Test yourself 139

Index 140
Acknowledgments 143
Test yourself: answers 144

How to use this book

This is an easy-to-follow guide to first aid that very clearly links theory to practice. The book features eight different sections, arranged by type of injury or condition. Throughout the book, there are realistic "incidents" photographed in the home, outdoors, or in the workplace that provide added realism and clearly show you what to do in an emergency. In addition, every section ends with a "Test yourself" panel to reinforce new learning. *Practical First Aid* also includes topics covered in the first-aid unit of the Public Service Award S/NVQ.

Emergency first-aid incidents
Each section of the book has a realistic incident showing how to put the guidance into practice

"What you should do" box outlines the first-aid action you should take in clearly identified steps

"Important" box highlights principal do's and don't's to enable you to give successful first aid

Captions around main picture help you identify first-aid priorities

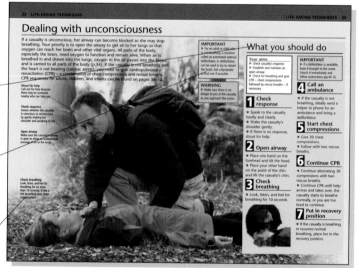

First-aid treatments
Every illness or injury is presented in a separate colour panel so that you can find information quickly and easily

"Your aims" and "You will need" boxes outline your treatment priorities and essential equipment

Step-by-step headings tell you exactly what you should do

"Signs and symptoms" help you confirm the casualty's injury

"Warning" box advises urgent action you may need to take

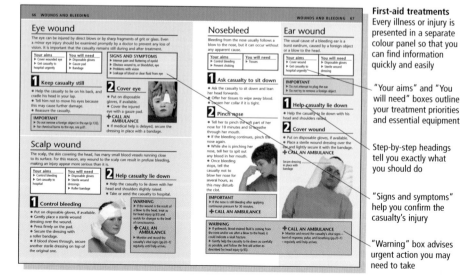

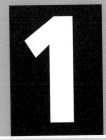

1 First-aid principles

This chapter explains the essentials that every first aider needs to know when dealing with an emergency. It sets out how to deal with every aspect of an incident, from the importance of ensuring your own and other people's safety to finding the best bandage or sling to put on an injury.

There are clear guidelines for dealing with any type of emergency, from rescuing a drowning casualty to managing a major incident with multiple casualties. Easy-to-follow charts and step-by-step instructions throughout show you how to assess a casualty's condition, summon help, and monitor a casualty while waiting for help to arrive.

Use the questionnaire on page 30 to test your understanding of your role as a first aider and your knowledge of first-aid materials.

Contents

Dealing with an incident	8
Assessing dangers	10
Avoiding cross-infection	13
Managing an incident	14
Coping with stress	15
Initial assessment of a casualty	16
Detailed assessment of a casualty	17
Carrying out a head-to-toe survey	18
Monitoring vital signs	20
First-aid materials	22
Sterile wound dressings	24
Plasters	25
Cold compresses	25
Roller bandages	26
Triangular bandages	27
Arm sling	28
Elevation sling	29
Test yourself	30

Dealing with an incident

Faced with an incident, first make sure that the area is safe, then assess any injuries; after that, decide what action to take. Whatever the situation, stay calm and confident to reassure the casualties. If you are sure that the scene of the incident is safe, try to locate all the casualties; some may have been thrown some distance or wandered away. If there is more than one casualty, decide who is the most seriously injured (see Dealing with more than one casualty p.14) and treat him first. Ask bystanders to help with the less seriously injured.

WARNING

▶ Make sure you are not putting yourself in danger when approaching an incident. If vehicles are involved, look in particular for smoke, fire, and hazardous chemicals (p.10).
▶ If there is an unconscious casualty, be ready to begin resuscitation if necessary (pp.36–52).

Make use of bystanders
Ask others for assistance, especially with calling for help, making the incident scene safe, and dealing with minor injuries

Make scene safe
At a car crash, put warning triangles 45m (150ft) away in each direction from the site of the incident

Listen to casualty
The casualty may be able to tell you what happened and how she is feeling

Attend seriously injured
Check the quiet casualty first as he may be unconscious

Check airway
If the casualty is unconscious, his airway may be blocked

Get help
Call the emergency services. Ideally, ask a bystander to do this

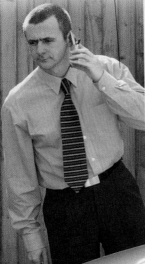

What you should do

Your aims
▶ Deal with any danger
▶ Assess incident
▶ Call emergency services
▶ Get help from others
▶ Give emergency aid

IMPORTANT
▶ If there are obvious dangers, wait for the emergency services to arrive – do not approach the scene until they tell you it is safe. Keep bystanders away.

1 Make area safe

● Check for danger as you approach the incident.
● If it is safe to do so, assess any casualties.
● If it is not safe, or if it is a major incident, such as a multiple car crash or a fire, call the emergency services.

2 Assess casualties

● Determine how many casualties are involved.
● Assess who is most seriously injured – attend to quiet casualties first as they may be unconscious.
● Carry out an initial assessment of the casualties (p.16).
● If any casualty is unconscious, be ready to begin resuscitation (pp.36–52).

3 Get help

● If any casualty is seriously injured, call an ambulance – tell the operator how many casualties there are.
● If possible, ask a bystander to make the call.

4 Give emergency aid

● If a casualty is conscious, carry out a detailed assessment (p.17).
● Treat life-threatening injuries such as severe bleeding before minor injuries such as sprains.
● Ask bystanders to help the less seriously injured or fetch necessary equipment.

5 Monitor casualties

● Monitor and record the casualties' vital signs – level of response, pulse, and breathing (pp.20–1) – regularly until help arrives.
● Pass the information you record onto the emergency services.

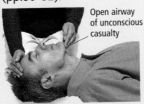

Open airway of unconscious casualty

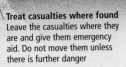

Treat casualties where found
Leave the casualties where they are and give them emergency aid. Do not move them unless there is further danger

Assessing dangers

In an emergency, you must make sure that by approaching an incident or a casualty, you are not putting your own life at risk. Stay calm, use common sense, take precautions to avoid the risk of cross-infection, and follow a plan to help you deal with casualties effectively.

Dealing with a traffic incident

At any traffic incident, you need to make the area safe before giving first aid. Make sure you are not putting yourself at risk by approaching the casualty when there is any danger. You need to protect yourself, any casualties, and other road users.

1 Call emergency services

- Park your vehicle, switch on your hazard lights, and alert the emergency services.

2 Warn others

- Set up warning triangles if possible. Place them in the road at least 45m (150ft) away in each direction from the site of the incident.
- Send helpers to warn other drivers.

3 Identify hazards

- Look for any hazards, such as vehicles with warning panels.
- Stabilise any vehicles by turning off the ignition and putting on the handbrake.

4 Check for casualties

- Check for casualties who may have been thrown some distance from a car or wandered away in shock.

Rescuing a casualty from water

Incidents around water often involve people who have fallen into, or have been swimming in, cold water or strong currents. Cold water can make swimming difficult or cause someone to swallow water. Do not endanger your own life when attempting a rescue.

1 Rescue from water's edge

- Lie down at the water's edge so that you do not get pulled into the water.
- Throw a rope or float to the casualty, or reach out with a stick or branch and pull him from the water.

2 If you have to go into water

- To make sure that you remain safe, wade rather than swim, and do not go out of your depth.
- Carefully lift the casualty out of the water.

3 Keep casualty warm

- Try to shield the casualty's body from wind to help prevent him from becoming any colder.
- Treat for hypothermia if necessary (p.86).
- Take or send the casualty to hospital, even if he appears to have recovered.
- If you are concerned, call an ambulance.

IMPORTANT
▶ If the casualty is unconscious, lift him out of the water and carry him with his head lower than his chest, which will stop fluid entering his airway if he vomits.

Electrical injuries

Injuries caused by electricity most commonly occur in the home as a result of contact with a low-voltage domestic current, usually due to faulty switches or appliances. Contact with electricity can cause serious injury or even death because the current passes through the body, causing burns and sometimes stopping the heart from beating. Contact with high-voltage electricity (below) is usually fatal.

1 Switch off current

● Break the electrical contact by switching off the current.

IMPORTANT
▶ Do not touch the casualty if he is still in contact with the electricity.

2 Separate casualty from electrical source

● If you cannot switch off the current, stand on some dry insulating material, such as a plastic mat, a folded newspaper, or a book such as a telephone directory.
● Using something wooden, push the casualty away from the source of the electricity or push the source away from the casualty. Do not use anything metallic.
● If it is still not possible to separate the casualty from the electrical source, loop some rope around his ankles and pull him away from the source.

Push electrical source away with a broom handle

WARNING
▶ If the casualty is unconscious, open the airway and check breathing. Put him in the recovery position if he is breathing. Be ready to begin resuscitation if necessary (pp.36–52).

✚ **CALL AN AMBULANCE**

3 Treat burns

● If the casualty is conscious, check for burns and treat accordingly (p.82).

Stand on a book to insulate yourself from electric current

High-voltage electricity

This is the type found in overhead power lines and high-tension cables. Anyone who survives contact will suffer serious burns.
● Call the emergency services.
● Ask for help from electrical engineers to shut off the power.
● Do not approach or allow anyone else to approach the casualty until you are certain that the power has been cut off and isolated. Everyone should stay at least 18m (60ft) away, as high-voltage electricity can jump ("arc") this distance.
● When it is safe to do so, assess the casualty.
● Be ready to begin resuscitation if necessary (pp.36–52).

Dealing with a fire

If a smoke alarm gives you warning of smoke or a fire, evacuate the building quickly. When fire breaks out, it is essential to think quickly and clearly because flames and smoke can spread rapidly. Alert the emergency services and warn anyone who may be in danger.

> **WARNING**
> ▶ Do not use lifts in any circumstances.
> ▶ Do not open a door without first touching the door or handle with the back of your hand to see if it is hot. Heat indicates fire behind the door, so choose a different escape route.

 Raise alarm

● In a public building, activate the nearest fire alarm and warn other people who are at risk.
● Call the emergency services.

2 Assess danger

● If the fire has taken hold, do not attempt to put it out yourself.
● If the fire is small, you discover it early, and you have a fire blanket or fire extinguisher, try to smother the flames. If you cannot extinguish the fire within 30 seconds, leave the building.

> **IMPORTANT**
> ▶ If trapped by fire, go into a room with a window and shut the door. Open the window and call for help. If escaping through a window, go out feet first. Lower yourself by your arms before dropping to the ground.

3 Get to safety

● If you are in a large building, follow the marked escape routes and help others, especially those who are vulnerable, such as children and elderly people.
● Close all doors behind you.
● Walk quickly and calmly – do not run.
● Do not enter a smoke-filled room.
● If you do need to cross a smoky area, try to stay close to the ground where the air will be clearer.

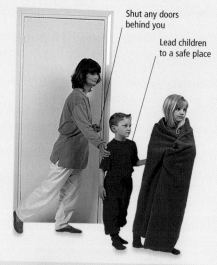

Shut any doors behind you

Lead children to a safe place

If a casualty's clothing is on fire

● Stop the casualty from running around.
● Drop him to the ground.
● Wrap him in heavy fabric, such as a wool or cotton blanket.
● Roll the casualty gently along the ground until the flames are extinguished.
● Do not use anything synthetic to try to put out the fire.

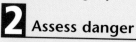

Use a thick rug to smother flames

Roll casualty gently until flames are out

Avoiding cross-infection

It is possible to be infected with certain viruses, such as HIV (human immunodeficiency virus) and hepatitis B or C, through contact with the blood or other body fluids of an infected person. Handle a casualty's body fluids as hygienically as possible to keep the risk of any cross-infection to a minimum. Avoid germs being transmitted when giving rescue breaths by using a special face shield (p.23). This is a plastic barrier with a filter that helps protect against contact with body fluids.

> **IMPORTANT**
> ▶ If gloves are unavailable, you must still give life-saving treatment.
> ▶ If your eyes, nose, mouth, or any wound on your skin is splashed by the casualty's blood, wash thoroughly with water immediately and consult a doctor as soon as possible.

Wash hands

Whenever possible, wash your hands thoroughly before and after treating a casualty. Make sure you wash the back and front of your hands.

Wear gloves

Whenever possible, put on disposable gloves. If you do not have any gloves, you can protect your hands with clean plastic bags.

Cover wound

When you cover a wound with a dressing, do not touch the inside sterile pad of the dressing. If possible, wear disposable gloves when applying dressings.

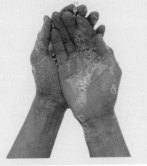
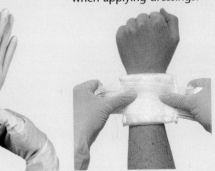

Removing waste

Once you have finished treatment, dispose of all waste carefully to prevent the spread of infection. Use plastic bags or, if you have them, special yellow biohazard bags. For sharp objects, use specially designed yellow boxes called sharps containers.

● Sharps containers are designed for the disposal of needles and any other sharp objects. They must be collected and disposed of by authorised waste collectors.

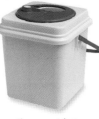

Sharps container

● Biohazard bags are designed for the disposal of soiled dressings and other waste products. They should be securely sealed and incinerated.

Keep gloves on while disposing of waste and then put them in bag

Disposal bag

Managing an incident

At the scene of a serious incident, it is vital to adopt a systematic approach, since there is likely to be panic and confusion. Make sure you are clear about how to deal with multiple casualties, get help from bystanders, and contact the emergency services.

Dealing with more than one casualty

In situations such as car crashes, you may find yourself dealing with several casualties at the same time. Whether you are working alone or with others, it is vital to stay calm.

1 Assess casualties

- Perform primary surveys (p.16) to identify casualties who have life-threatening injuries.
- Check quiet casualties first; they may be unconscious.
- Enlist help to get casualties with minor injuries quickly from the site and allow access to serious cases.

2 Attend to unconscious casualties

- Prioritise the treatment of any unconscious casualties.

3 Treat conscious casualties

- Treat conscious casualties with serious injuries.
- Treat casualties with minor injuries.

Moving a casualty

- Do not move a casualty to give first aid unless he is in immediate danger, it is safe for you to approach, and you have the correct training and equipment.

- You may need to move a casualty if: he is in danger of drowning; he is at risk due to fire, smoke, a bomb, or gunfire; or he is in or near a collapsing building.

Getting help from others

You may be faced with several tasks at the scene of the incident, such as maintaining safety, calling for help, and starting first aid. Bystanders may be able to assist you.

1 Give clear instructions

- Let everyone know at the scene of an incident that you are trained in first aid.
- Be clear with bystanders about what you want them to do.
- You may want to ask bystanders to: locate casualties; call the emergency services; control traffic and onlookers; bring first-aid equipment; maintain a casualty's privacy; or help with first aid.

2 Follow through

- If you do send a bystander to telephone for help, see that he returns to confirm that the call has been made.
- If other first aiders come forward, give them as much information as possible. The most senior first aider present should take charge of the team.
- When the emergency services arrive, the senior officer will take control.

Getting appropriate help

Help in an emergency is available from the following sources:

- Emergency services – police, fire, and ambulance services, and mine, mountain, cave, fell rescue, and coastguard. Dial 999 free from any phone in the UK, or the European Union emergency number 112.
- Health services – doctor, nurse, midwife, dentist, or NHS Direct (NHS24 in Scotland), a 24-hour UK-based medical advice service.
- Utilities – gas, electricity, and water.

Throughout this book, advice is given on the type of medical help to seek. There are three main categories as follows:

✚ GET MEDICAL HELP
when advice about treatment is necessary.

✚ TAKE OR SEND CASUALTY TO HOSPITAL
when hospital treatment is essential. You may be able to take the casualty yourself.

✚ CALL AN AMBULANCE
when urgent treatment is needed.

Calling the emergency services

When you dial 999, you will be asked which service you need. If there are casualties, ask for an ambulance. Give the operator the following details:
- Your telephone number.
- The location of the incident.
- The type and seriousness of the incident, for example, "One car overturned, two casualties trapped".
- The number of casualties and details of injury, for example, "One male with breathing difficulties – has an inhaler".
- Details of hazards such as chemicals.

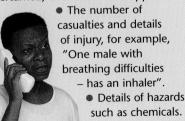

Coping with stress

An emergency can be very distressing for everyone involved. To safeguard your own welfare and remain effective as a first aider, recognise that feelings of stress are normal.

1 Be prepared for reaction

- Realise that it is natural to feel stressed about giving first aid and to be emotional after you have finished treating a casualty.
- You might feel satisfied at having done a good job, confused about whether you did the "right things", or angry and sad if the outcome of the incident is upsetting.

2 Watch for symptoms

- Stress may manifest itself in any of the following symptoms: tremor of the hands and stomach; excessive sweating; flashbacks; nightmares or disturbed sleep; tearfulness; tension and irritability; or a feeling of withdrawal and isolation.

3 Talk about feelings

- To help you face up to your emotions, talk about how you feel with a friend or colleague. By releasing your feelings as soon after the event as possible, you should find yourself able to cope more easily.

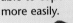

IMPORTANT
▶ If you are experiencing symptoms of stress and they do not pass in time, or if you are concerned, seek further advice from your doctor.

Initial assessment of a casualty

Your priority when attending a casualty is to assess him for life-threatening conditions, such as lack of breathing, that need urgent first aid. Carry out a more detailed assessment (opposite) only when you have established that the casualty is breathing normally.

Primary survey

This intial assessment involves looking for danger to yourself and the casualty, checking whether the casualty is conscious and breathing (and beginning cardiopulmonary resuscitation – CPR – if necessary). Detailed guidelines for life-saving sequences for adults, children, and infants can be found on pages 36–52.

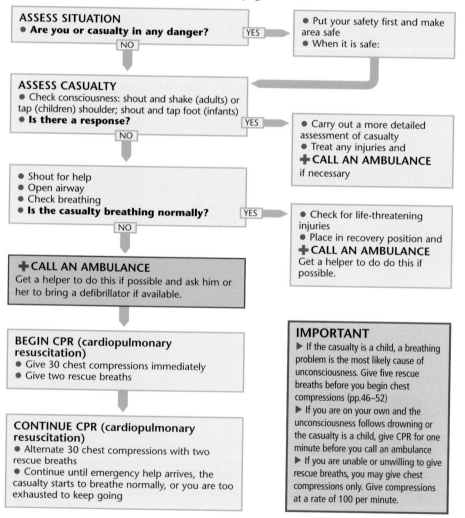

ASSESS SITUATION
- **Are you or casualty in any danger?**   YES   NO

- Put your safety first and make area safe
- When it is safe:

ASSESS CASUALTY
- Check consciousness: shout and shake (adults) or tap (children) shoulder; shout and tap foot (infants)
- **Is there a response?**   YES   NO

- Carry out a more detailed assessment of casualty
- Treat any injuries and
✚ **CALL AN AMBULANCE**
if necessary

- Shout for help
- Open airway
- Check breathing
- **Is the casualty breathing normally?**   YES   NO

- Check for life-threatening injuries
- Place in recovery position and
✚ **CALL AN AMBULANCE**
Get a helper to do do this if possible.

✚ **CALL AN AMBULANCE**
Get a helper to do this if possible and ask him or her to bring a defibrillator if available.

BEGIN CPR (cardiopulmonary resuscitation)
- Give 30 chest compressions immediately
- Give two rescue breaths

CONTINUE CPR (cardiopulmonary resuscitation)
- Alternate 30 chest compressions with two rescue breaths
- Continue until emergency help arrives, the casualty starts to breathe normally, or you are too exhausted to keep going

IMPORTANT
▶ If the casualty is a child, a breathing problem is the most likely cause of unconsciousness. Give five rescue breaths before you begin chest compressions (pp.46–52)
▶ If you are on your own and the unconsciousness follows drowning or the casualty is a child, give CPR for one minute before you call an ambulance
▶ If you are unable or unwilling to give rescue breaths, you may give chest compressions only. Give compressions at a rate of 100 per minute.

Detailed assessment of a casualty

Once the casualty is out of danger, you have completed the primary survey, and no further life-saving actions are needed, carry out a detailed assessment of the casualty, known as a secondary survey, to find out more about the casualty's condition. If a casualty complains of a particular problem, treat this first. You also need to monitor the casualty's vital signs – level of response, pulse, and breathing (pp.20–21).

> **Your aims**
> ▶ Obtain full history of incident by questioning casualty or onlookers
> ▶ Find out more about circumstances in which injury was sustained and forces involved – this is known as the mechanics of injury
> ▶ Assess general signs and symptoms – find out how casualty is feeling and how serious his condition is
> ▶ Examine casualty thoroughly – look for details of casualty's condition that you can see, feel, hear, or smell

Taking a history of the incident

Try to form a full picture of the situation by asking the following questions:

● **What happened?**
How did the problem occur? Has the casualty had this problem before? Does anything make it better or worse?
● **When did it happen?**
What time did the problem start? Was the casualty doing anything in particular?
● **Where did it happen?**
Was the casualty in a particular environment when the problem started? Were there any hazards in the area?

● **Why did it happen?**
Does the casualty know why it happened? Were there any factors in the area that might have contributed to the problem?

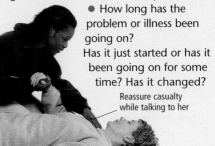

● **How long has the problem or illness been going on?**
Has it just started or has it been going on for some time? Has it changed?

Reassure casualty while talking to her

Finding out how the incident happened

You may be able to gain more clues about potential injuries by looking to see how an incident has happened. For example:
● If a casualty falls from a height of over 2m (6ft), he is likely to sustain severe injuries, such as pelvic fractures, spinal injuries, and damage to internal organs.
● In a car crash, a casualty who is hit from the side is likely to sustain more severe injuries than if he is hit from the front. This is because the side of the car provides less protection.

● If a driver is wearing a seatbelt and the vehicle is struck head-on or from behind, this may result in a whiplash injury, with strained muscles and sprained ligaments in the neck. There may also be bruising due to seatbelt restraint.
● If a casualty dives into the shallow end of a swimming pool and hits his head, he is likely to sustain a neck injury.
● If a casualty is thrown from a horse at speed and hits his head, he is likely to also have a neck injury.

Carrying out a head-to-toe survey

It is important to examine a casualty from head to toe to assess the seriousness of her injuries. Signs and symptoms may change while you are looking after a casualty. In addition, monitor her vital signs – level of response, pulse, and breathing (pp.20–1) – regularly. Look for clues, listen to what she says, feel for anything abnormal, and smell for anything unusual. Work along the body carefully, while talking reassuringly to the casualty to calm her. Ask any questions that could be relevant to her condition.

1 Look for general signs and symptoms

- Ask the casualty if she feels any pain and, if so, where.
- Feel her skin – it may be cold, clammy, hot, or sweaty.
- Watch her skin for blueness (cyanosis), especially around the lips.
- Check her breathing – it may be rapid, slow, shallow, or laboured.
- Feel her pulse – it may be fast, slow, weak, or erratic.
- Watch the casualty's level of response – she may be drowsy, confused, or anxious.

2 Examine head and neck

- Run your hands carefully over the casualty's head. If you suspect a neck injury, be careful not to move the head. Feel for signs of any blood, swelling, or a depression in the skull – these are all signs of a skull fracture.
- Speak clearly into each ear and watch for the response.
- Look for any blood or a yellowish fluid coming from either ear or from the nose – these are signs of a skull fracture.
- Look for bleeding, bruising, swelling, or a foreign object in the eye. Ask if the casualty can see clearly.
- Look to see if the casualty's pupils are equal in size and constrict in response to light. If they are unequal in size, this could indicate cerebral compression.
- Look for bleeding, bruising, or swelling around the mouth.
- Detect any unpleasant odours on the breath by smelling near to the mouth.
- Loosen clothing at the neck and look for a hole (stoma) in the windpipe left by a surgical operation, or a medical warning necklace.
- Ask the casualty if she has any neck pain. Feel the collarbones for deformity.

Looking for external clues

If a casualty is unable to cooperate, look for the following clues:
- Objects that may have caused injury.
- Objects that may indicate the problem, such as used needles and syringes, alcohol bottles, or tins of glue.
- Medicines that may indicate the medical condition of the casualty.
- An inhaler that may indicate asthma.
- An auto-injector that may indicate a risk of anaphylactic shock.
- A warning bracelet that gives a phone number to ring for information about the casualty's medical history.
- A card that indicates a history of allergy, diabetes, or epilepsy.
- A special bracelet, necklace, card, or medallion carrying medical information.

3 Check chest and abdomen

- Look for any wounds to the chest, or abnormal movement.
- Ask the casualty to take a deep breath and look to see if her chest expands evenly and equally on both sides – if not, this may indicate a chest injury.
- Listen for coughing or wheezing, as this may indicate asthma.
- Feel the ribcage for swelling, deformity, or tenderness.
- Look for wounds, bruising, or swelling of the abdomen.
- Feel for any tenderness or rigidity of the muscles – signs of an internal injury.

- Look at the clothing for signs of incontinence or bleeding from orifices.
- Feel the pelvis for any deformity.

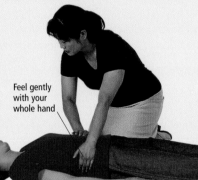

Feel gently with your whole hand

4 Assess whether there is back pain

- If the casualty complains of severe back pain or difficulty moving the limbs, suspect a back injury and do not move the casualty.

- Ask about numbness or tingling.
- If the casualty has no sign of injury, ask if there is a previous history of back pain.

5 Look at arms and hands

- Look for any bleeding, bruising, swelling, or deformity.
- Ask the casualty to move her arms at the different joints.
- Look for any needle marks or a medical warning device.
- Check the colour of the fingers – if they are blue, this may indicate a problem with blood circulation or an injury due to cold.

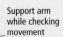

Support arm while checking movement

6 Check legs and feet

- Look for any bleeding, bruising, swelling, or deformity.
- Ask the casualty to move the legs at the different joints.

- Check the colour of her feet and toes – if they are blue, this may indicate a problem with blood circulation or an injury due to cold.

Monitoring vital signs

While you are waiting for an ambulance, it is important to keep monitoring the casualty's level of response, pulse, and breathing. These vital signs will help you assess whether his condition is stable, worsening, or improving, or whether there are any specific problems. You may also need to check his body temperature. Write down your findings and the intervals between each assessment and give the information to medical staff or the emergency services.

Checking level of response

To help you assess a casualty's level of consciousness, use the AVPU code. Follow this code at regular intervals, so that you can check whether the casualty's condition is improving or deteriorating.
● A – Is the casualty **Alert** and responding to you normally? This means that he is fully conscious.

● V – Does the casualty respond to your **Voice**, answer simple questions, and obey simple commands?
● P – Does the casualty respond to **Pain**?
● U – Is the casualty **Unresponsive** to everything? This means that he is unconscious. Be ready to begin resuscitation if necessary (pp.36–52).

Checking pulse

● The normal pulse rate in adults is 60–80 beats per minute. In very fit young adults the pulse is slower and in children it is much faster – up to 140 beats per minute.
● Check a casualty's pulse at the neck (carotid pulse) or at the wrist (radial pulse). In infants, the easiest pulse to find is the brachial pulse in the upper arm.

● When checking a casualty's pulse, use your fingers rather than your thumb (which has its own pulse) and press lightly downwards in order to feel the beat.
● Using a watch, monitor and write down the following details: rate (the number of beats per minute); strength (whether the pulse is strong or weak); rhythm (whether the pulse is regular or irregular).

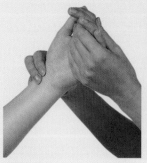

Radial pulse
Place two or three fingers just below the wrist creases at the base of the thumb. Use the pads of the fingers to improve sensitivity.

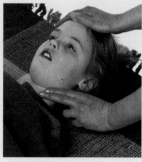

Carotid pulse
Place two fingers on the side of the casualty's neck, in the hollow between the windpipe and the large neck muscle.

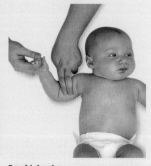

Brachial pulse
Place two fingers on the inner side of an infant's upper arm midway between the shoulder and elbow. Use the pads of the fingers to improve sensitivity.

Checking breathing rate

● The normal breathing rate in adults is 12–16 breaths and in young children 20–30 breaths per minute.
● Listen to the casualty's breaths, watch his chest rise and fall, and count the number of breaths in 1 minute.
● For young children, put your hand on the chest and feel for breathing.
● Listen carefully for any breathing difficulties or unusual noises.
● Using a watch, monitor and write down the following details: rate (number of breaths per minute); depth (deep or shallow breaths); quality (easy, difficult, or painful breaths); noise (quiet or noisy breathing).

Place hand on child's chest and feel for breaths

Measuring temperature

● Normal body temperature is around 37°C (98.6°F). A high temperature is usually caused by infection; a low temperature (see Hypothermia p.86) may result from exposure to cold and/or wet weather conditions.
● To obtain an accurate temperature reading use a thermometer.
● There are several types of thermometer, including glass mercury, digital, forehead, and aural. Whichever type you have, make sure you know how to use it.
● A glass mercury thermometer can be used to measure temperature under the tongue or in the armpit. Check the mercury level is below 37°C (98.6°F) before use and leave the thermometer in place for 2–3 minutes before reading.

● A digital thermometer can be used under the tongue or in the armpit. Leave it in place for about 30 seconds until it "beeps"; then read the display.
● A forehead thermometer is useful for measuring temperature in a young child. Hold the small, heat-sensitive strip against the forehead for about 30 seconds and its colour will change to show the temperature.
● An ear sensor, or aural thermometer, is useful for a sick child. Place its tip inside the ear to get a reading within 1 second.

WARNING
▶ Never put a digital or mercury thermometer in the mouth of a child under 7. There is a risk that he or she may bite on it and break it.

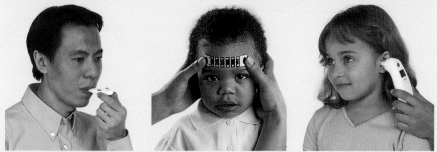

Digital thermometer　　　　Forehead thermometer　　　　Aural thermometer

First-aid materials

Keep an easily identifiable first-aid kit in a safe, accessible place at home. If you have a car, keep a kit in it. Put it under a seat or in the boot – never on the back shelf as it may fly off and cause an injury if you have to brake suddenly. You can buy a first-aid kit or assemble items yourself and store them in a clean, waterproof container. Dressings and bandages form the basis of a home first-aid kit, but there are a few useful extras (opposite). Check all equipment regularly and replace used or out-of-date items.

Bandages

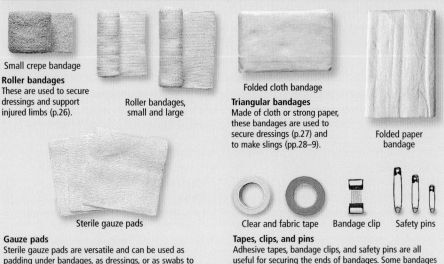

Small crepe bandage

Roller bandages
These are used to secure dressings and support injured limbs (p.26).

Roller bandages, small and large

Folded cloth bandage

Triangular bandages
Made of cloth or strong paper, these bandages are used to secure dressings (p.27) and to make slings (pp.28–9).

Folded paper bandage

Sterile gauze pads

Gauze pads
Sterile gauze pads are versatile and can be used as padding under bandages, as dressings, or as swabs to clean around wounds.

Clear and fabric tape   Bandage clip   Safety pins

Tapes, clips, and pins
Adhesive tapes, bandage clips, and safety pins are all useful for securing the ends of bandages. Some bandages come with a clip attached.

Tying a reef knot

Always use a reef knot to secure a bandage or sling because it will not slip and it is also easy to undo. Since the knot lies flat against the casualty, it is more comfortable. Follow the sequence below for tying a reef knot.

● Hold one end of the bandage in each hand. Take the right end of the bandage over the left.

● Pass what is now the left end under and through the gap.
● Take what is now the right end over the left. Pass it through the gap and pull the knot tight to secure it.

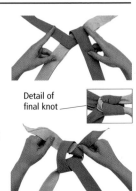

Detail of final knot

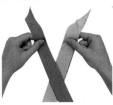

Dressings

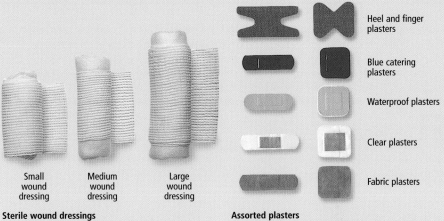

Heel and finger plasters

Blue catering plasters

Waterproof plasters

Clear plasters

Fabric plasters

Small wound dressing

Medium wound dressing

Large wound dressing

Sterile wound dressings
These dressings are sealed and come with an attached bandage, and in various sizes. They are placed on wounds to help control bleeding and prevent infection.

Assorted plasters
These adhesive dressings, made of fabric or waterproof plastic, are used to cover small cuts and grazes. People who work with food have to use blue plasters.

Useful additions to a first-aid kit

Plastic face shield

Wound cleansing wipes

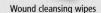

Scissors   Tweezers   Notepad and pencil

For protection
Disposable gloves should be worn whenever you come into contact with body fluids, such as blood. A face shield placed over a casualty's mouth will protect you and the casualty from infections when giving rescue breaths. Use wound cleansing wipes to clean the skin around wounds and to clean your hands if you have no soap and water.

Plastic disposable gloves

Household items
There are a few household items that are useful to keep in a first-aid kit, such as scissors, tweezers, and a notepad and pencil or pen.

Foil survival bag

Plastic survival bag

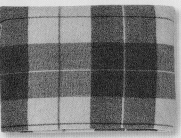

Blanket

Warning triangle

For outdoors
A camping or car first-aid kit could include a blanket and a survival bag. You could also store a warning triangle in the car boot for placing in the road at the site of a car crash.

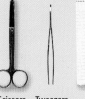

Sterile wound dressings

These absorbent gauze pads have been sterilised and individually sealed in protective wrapping. As soon as the protective wrapping is taken off, the dressing is no longer sterile. Make sure the dressing pad is large enough to extend beyond the edges of the wound. If any blood shows through after the dressing is secure, do not remove the dressing but place another one on top. If blood seeps through the second dressing, remove both dressings and start again. If the dressing does not have an attached bandage, place the pad over the injury and secure it in place with a separate bandage.

1 Unroll dressing

- Put on disposable gloves, if available.
- Unwrap the dressing and unroll the short end of the bandage until the end of the dressing pad is visible.
- Holding the bandage, open the pad next to the wound and place on the wound.

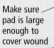

Make sure pad is large enough to cover wound

Hold bandage on either side of pad

IMPORTANT
▶ Do not slide the pad onto the wound. Position it carefully over the wound.
▶ Do not touch the gauze side of the pad.

2 Bandage over pad

- Hold the sterile pad in place on the injury and use the long end of the roller bandage to secure the pad by winding it around the affected body part.
- Make sure the bandage covers the whole of the pad.

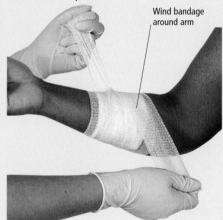

Wind bandage around arm

3 Secure bandage

- Tie the ends of the bandages in a reef knot (p.22) over the pad.
- Check the circulation in the hand (p.26). If the bandage is too tight, loosen it and reapply.

Plasters

These adhesive dressings are used to cover small cuts and grazes. Ask the casualty if he is allergic to plasters before applying one. If he is, use a sterile dressing instead.

1 Open plaster pack

● Wash your hands and then open the sterile pack.

2 Put plaster on wound

● Taking care not to touch the pad in the centre, gently pull back the plastic covers until the dressing pad is exposed.
● Place the dressing pad on the wound and pull the plastic covers further back until the plaster is secured in place.

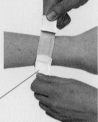

Pull back
plastic covers

Emergency dressings

If you do not have sterile wound dressings or plasters, you can use any piece of clean, non-fluffy material, such as a handkerchief.
● Wash your hands, hold the material by the corners, and let it fall open.
● Fold the material to the desired size so what was the inside surface, and probably cleaner, is now on the outside.
● Holding the material at the edges, place it over the wound and secure in place with a bandage, tape, or a scarf.
● If you have neither dressings nor material, cover the wound with a clean polythene bag or any clean item found in the kitchen, such as kitchen roll or polythene film.

Cold compresses

These are used to reduce bruising and swelling, which helps relieve pain. Apply for 10 minutes and then reassess the injury. You should reapply the cold compress at 10-minute intervals for up to 30 minutes, if necessary.

1 Wet a cloth

● Soak a face cloth, thin towel, or similar piece of material in cold water, then wring it out until it stops dripping.

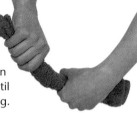

2 Position pad over injury

● Fold the cloth to the required size and place it over the injury. If possible, replace the pad every 10 minutes, or cool it by dripping cold water onto it.

Using an ice pack

A plastic bag containing ice cubes or a bag of frozen peas or sweetcorn makes a very effective cold compress.
● Fill a plastic bag half to two-thirds full of ice cubes.
● Squeeze the air out of the bag and seal it.
● Wrap the bag in a thin towel and place it over the casualty's injury. Apply for 10 minutes and replace as necessary.

IMPORTANT
▶ Do not put ice directly onto the skin because it will burn.

Roller bandages

Use a roller bandage to support muscle or joint injuries, secure dressings, or to apply pressure to control bleeding. Once the bandage is secured, check the circulation in the fingers or toes beyond the bandage by pressing the skin until it turns pale and watching for colour to return. If the colour does not return, loosen the bandage.

1 Bandage around limb

- Place the end of the bandage on the limb and make a firm, straight turn to secure the bandage. Keep the injured part supported as you do so.

Wind bandage around limb

2 Work up limb

- Working up the limb, make a series of spiral turns with the bandage, allowing each successive turn to cover two-thirds of the previous one.

Work up limb

3 Secure bandage

- Finish winding with a straight turn.
- Secure the end with a safety pin, bandage clip, or tape. Alternatively, tuck in the remaining bandage.

Secure bandage

Bandaging an ankle or hand

To support an ankle or hand injury, you need to adapt the bandaging technique. Extend the bandage well beyond the injury so that pressure is applied over the entire injured area. When bandaging a hand, start at the wrist and leave the thumb free.

1 Bandage around ankle

- Wind the bandage around the ankle and take it diagonally across the foot.
- Bring the bandage under the ball of the foot to the base of the big toe.

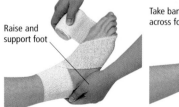

Raise and support foot

2 Bandage across foot

- Pass the bandage across the top of the casualty's foot and back around the ankle.
- Make another straight turn around the ankle.

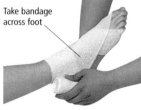

Take bandage across foot

3 Secure bandage

- Continue figure-of-eight turns around the foot and ankle until they are covered.
- Make a final turn around the ankle and secure at the ankle as described above.

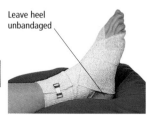

Leave heel unbandaged

Triangular bandages

Use a triangular bandage to make slings and to secure injured limbs. Although they are usually made from unbleached calico, you can make one yourself from similar material about 1m (3ft) square cut diagonally in half. The bandage can be folded in two ways: broad-fold and narrow-fold. A broad-fold bandage is used mainly to immobilise and support a limb; a narrow-fold bandage is most commonly used to immobilise feet and ankles.

Open triangular bandage

1 Broad-fold bandage

- Lay the bandage on a flat, clean surface, and fold the point of the triangular bandage to the base.
- Fold the bandage in half again.

Broad-fold bandage

2 Narrow-fold bandage

- Fold a broad-fold bandage in half along its length.

Narrow-fold bandage

Cover bandages

A triangular bandage can also be used to hold a light dressing in place, especially on a hand or foot – but it is not suitable for controlling bleeding.

1 Fold bandage over hand

- Place the casualty's hand on the bandage.
- Bring the point of the bandage over the hand onto the forearm.

Fold point of bandage over hand

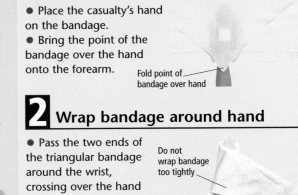

2 Wrap bandage around hand

- Pass the two ends of the triangular bandage around the wrist, crossing over the hand in opposite directions.

Do not wrap bandage too tightly

3 Tie ends together

- Tie the two ends together in a reef knot (p.22) above the point of the bandage.
- Gently pull the point of the bandage down to tighten and secure the bandage over the dressing.

Knot lies flat on limb

Detail of knot

4 Secure bandage

- Lift the point of the bandage over the reef knot. Tuck in the point or secure it over the reef knot with a safety pin.

Cover knot with point of bandage

Detail of tuck

Arm sling

Use an arm sling to support an injured upper arm, forearm, or wrist and to immobilise an arm if there is a chest injury. Like the elevation sling (opposite), an arm sling should be used only if the casualty is able to bend his elbow.

You will need
▶ Triangular bandage
▶ Safety pin

IMPORTANT
▶ Keep the injured arm well supported until the sling is secure and supports the arm itself.

1 Support injured arm

● Sit the casualty down and ask him to support the injured arm with his other arm.
● Slide one end of a triangular bandage through the hollow under his elbow.
● Pull the upper end until it rests by the collarbone on the side of the injury.

Pull bandage around back of neck

Get casualty to support injured arm

2 Secure sling

● Bring the lower end of the bandage up over the forearm so that it supports the injured arm.
● Tie a reef knot (p.22) in the hollow above the collarbone on the injured side.
● Tuck the ends of the bandage under the reef knot.

Bring lower end of bandage over arm

3 Pin bandage at elbow

● Tuck the excess bandage behind the elbow and secure the point with either a safety pin (below) or a twist (opposite).

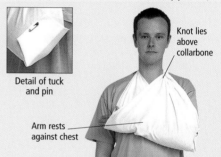

Detail of tuck and pin

Knot lies above collarbone

Arm rests against chest

Improvising an arm sling

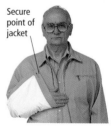

Secure point of jacket

● For a zip-up jacket, turn the open jacket up over the arm and attach it to the top of the jacket with a safety pin.

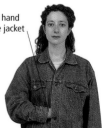

Place hand inside jacket

● For a button-up jacket, place the casualty's hand inside the jacket between its fastenings.

Elevation sling

Use this type of sling to support the arm in a raised position when a hand or forearm is injured and bleeding needs to be controlled, to support a broken hand, to reduce swelling, and to support the arm in the event of a broken collarbone or rib.

You will need
▶ Triangular bandage
▶ Safety pin

IMPORTANT
▶ Keep the injured arm well supported until the sling is secure and supports the arm itself.

1 Support injured arm

● Sit the casualty down and ask her to support her arm across the chest so that the fingers reach the opposite shoulder.

Support arm at elbow

2 Position bandage

● Lay a triangular bandage over her arm with one end over the shoulder, making sure the point is past the elbow.

Lay bandage across arm

Longest edge of bandage

3 Tuck in bandage

● Tuck the base of the bandage under the casualty's forearm and elbow.
● Take the lower end of the bandage around the casualty's back and up towards the other shoulder.

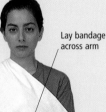

Tuck in excess bandage

Arm is now supported by bandage

4 Secure sling

● Tie both ends of the bandage together in the hollow above the collarbone using a reef knot (p.22).
● Secure the point of the bandage with a safety pin (opposite). If you do not have a pin, twist the point of the bandage and tuck it in above the elbow (below).
● Check the circulation in the thumb (p.26).

Detail of twist

Improvising an elevation sling

● A turned-up jumper can be used to support an arm.

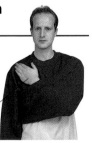

Secure hand against shoulder

Test yourself

Now that you have read and studied the chapter on first-aid principles, see if you can answer the questions below. After completing the questions, check your answers against the correct ones on page 144.

1 What should you do first when arriving at the scene of an incident?
....
....

2 What should you do if there is a major incident such as a fire?
....
....

3 When dealing with several casualties at the same time, which ones should you tend to first?
....
....

4 What should you wear if you are likely to come into contact with body fluids such as blood?
....

5 What is a sharps container?
....
....

6 How do you get in touch with the emergency services?
....
....

7 When checking level of response, what does AVPU stand for?
A ....
V ....
P ....
U ....

8 Where on the body can you feel the pulse?
....
....

9 Which of the following are basic items for a first-aid kit?
a Sterile wound dressings .... ☐
b Blanket .... ☐
c Triangular bandage .... ☐
d Plasters .... ☐
e Scissors .... ☐
f Safety pins .... ☐

10 Why is a reef knot a good way to secure a bandage?
....
....

11 Why should you not put ice directly onto the skin?
....
....

12 How do you check that a bandage on a hand or foot is not too tight?
....
....

13 For what reasons would you use an arm sling and an elevation sling?
Arm sling ....
....
....
Elevation sling ....
....
....
....

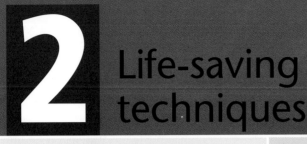

2 Life-saving techniques

To stay alive, the body needs a continuous supply of oxygen. This chapter shows you how to maintain the supply of oxygen for a casualty who is not breathing. It provides an up-to-date guide to the life-saving techniques used to treat casualties who are unconscious or choking.

Easy-to-understand anatomical information explains how the breathing and blood circulation systems work, to help you understand why the resuscitation techniques are effective. The methods used vary for adults, children, and infants so there are separate life-saving sequences for each.

This chapter includes instructions for using an automated external defibrillator (also known as an AED or a defibrillator), a machine that can be used to treat a casualty whose heart has stopped beating.

Once you have studied this chapter, use the questionnaire on page 56 to test your knowledge and understanding of the procedures described here.

Contents

Dealing with unconsciousness	32
Breathing and blood circulation	34
How resuscitation works	35
Resuscitation techniques	36
Check response (adult)	37
Check breathing (adult)	37
Recovery position (adult)	38
Rescue breathing (adult)	40
CPR (adult)	42
Using a defibrillator	44
Check response (child)	46
Check breathing (child)	46
Recovery position (child)	47
Rescue breathing (child)	48
CPR (child)	49
Check response (infant)	50
Check breathing (infant)	50
Recovery position (infant)	51
Rescue breathing (infant)	51
CPR (infant)	52
Choking (adult)	53
Choking (child)	54
Choking (infant)	55
Test yourself	56

Dealing with unconsciousness

If a casualty is unconscious, her airway can become blocked so she may stop breathing. Your priority is to open the airway to get air to her lungs so that oxygen can reach her brain and other vital organs. All parts of the body, especially the brain, need oxygen to function and remain alive. When air is breathed in and drawn into the lungs, oxygen in the air passes into the blood and is carried to all parts of the body (p.34). If the casualty is not breathing and the heart is not beating (cardiac arrest), you need to give cardiopulmonary resuscitation (CPR) – a combination of chest compressions and rescue breaths. CPR sequences for adults, children, and infants can be found on pages 36–52.

Shout for help
Call out for help because there may be someone nearby who can help you

Check response
Assess whether the casualty is conscious or unconscious by gently shaking her shoulder and speaking to her

Open airway
Make sure the casualty's airway is open to allow an unobstructed passage of air to the lungs

Check breathing
Look, listen, and feel for breathing for no more than 10 seconds. If she is not breathing normally, start chest compressions

IMPORTANT
▶ For an adult or child who is not breathing, a machine called an automated external defibrillator, or defibrillator, can be used to try to restart the heart. Ask a bystander to find one if possible.

WARNING
▶ Make sure there is no danger to you or the casualty as you approach the scene.

What you should do

Your aims
▶ Check casualty's response
▶ Establish and maintain an open airway
▶ Check for breathing and give CPR – chest compressions followed by rescue breaths – if necessary

IMPORTANT
▶ If a defibrillator is available, have it brought to the scene. Attach it immediately and follow instructions (pp.44–5).

1 Check response

- Speak to the casualty loudly and clearly.
- Shake the casualty's shoulder gently.
- If there is no response, shout for help.

2 Open airway

- Place one hand on the forehead and tilt the head.
- Place your other hand on the point of the chin and lift the casualty's chin.

3 Check breathing

- Look, listen, and feel for breathing for 10 seconds.

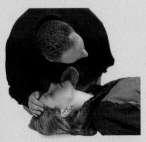

4 Call an ambulance

- If the casualty is not breathing, ideally send a helper to phone for an ambulance and bring a defibrillator.

5 Start chest compressions

- Give 30 chest compressions.
- Follow with two rescue breaths.

6 Continue CPR

- Continue alternating 30 compressions with two rescue breaths.
- Continue CPR until help arrives and takes over, the casualty starts to breathe normally, or you are too tired to continue.

7 Put in recovery position

- If the casualty is breathing or resumes normal breathing, place her in the recovery position.

Breathing and blood circulation

Oxygen is essential to life – every cell in the body needs it to be able to function. If deprived of oxygen for any length of time, the cells die – those in the brain survive only minutes without an adequate supply. Oxygen is taken in when we breathe in via the airway and the lungs (respiratory system). It is then transported around the body by the heart and blood vessels (circulatory system).

How the body gets oxygen

As we breathe in, muscles in the chest wall and diaphragm contract, the chest cavity enlarges, and air containing oxygen enters the body through the mouth and nose and passes into the windpipe, or airway. The airway divides into two smaller tubes (bronchi), one for each lung. In the lungs, the bronchi divide into smaller tubes called bronchioles that end in microscopic air sacs (alveoli). Oxygen from the air we breathe in passes through the walls of these air sacs into small blood vessels (capillaries), where it is picked up by the blood. The oxygen-rich blood is then carried to the heart and pumped around the body. When we breathe out, the muscles in the chest wall and diaphragm relax, the chest cavity contracts, and the lungs shrink, sending used air up the airway and out of the body.

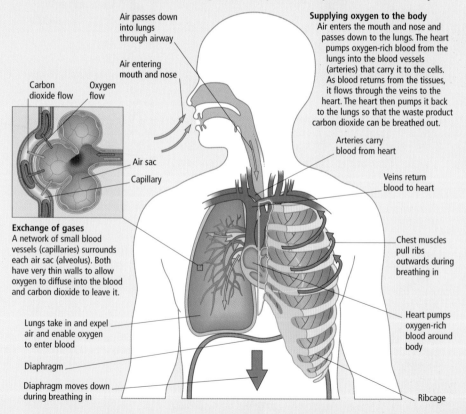

Air passes down into lungs through airway

Air entering mouth and nose

Carbon dioxide flow

Oxygen flow

Air sac

Capillary

Supplying oxygen to the body
Air enters the mouth and nose and passes down to the lungs. The heart pumps oxygen-rich blood from the lungs into the blood vessels (arteries) that carry it to the cells. As blood returns from the tissues, it flows through the veins to the heart. The heart then pumps it back to the lungs so that the waste product carbon dioxide can be breathed out.

Arteries carry blood from heart

Veins return blood to heart

Exchange of gases
A network of small blood vessels (capillaries) surrounds each air sac (alveolus). Both have very thin walls to allow oxygen to diffuse into the blood and carbon dioxide to leave it.

Chest muscles pull ribs outwards during breathing in

Lungs take in and expel air and enable oxygen to enter blood

Diaphragm

Diaphragm moves down during breathing in

Heart pumps oxygen-rich blood around body

Ribcage

How resuscitation works

With an unconscious casualty, breathing and circulation may not function properly, so the body's cells are starved of oxygen. The possibility of recovery decreases rapidly, within a few minutes. By using cardiopulmonary resuscitation (CPR), which involves keeping the casualty's airway open, giving him chest compressions to keep blood circulating and rescue breaths to imitate breathing, you can supply oxygen to the casualty until emergency aid arrives. This is easy to remember as the ABC of resuscitation – A is for airway, B for breathing, and C for chest compressions. A machine called a defibrillator can be used to restart the heart (p.44).

Agonal breathing is common in the first few minutes after a heart stops (cardiac arrest). It is usually in the form of infrequent short gasps for breath. If present it should not be mistaken for normal breathing and you should start CPR without hesitation.

Opening the airway

Loss of muscle control in an unconscious casualty, can cause the tongue to fall back and block the airway. When this happens, breathing becomes difficult and noisy, or impossible. Tilting the head back and lifting the chin lifts the tongue, allowing the casualty to breathe.

Maintaining circulation

If the heart stops beating, oxygenated blood does not circulate around the body and oxygen cannot reach the vital organs, such as the brain. Chest compressions act as a mechanical aid to get some blood flowing around the body. Pushing vertically down on the centre of the chest squeezes the chest and heart, forcing blood around the body. As pressure is released, the chest rises, which allows replacement blood to flow into the chest.

Pushing down on chest using correct technique can keep blood circulating

Breathing for a casualty

The air that we breathe out contains about 16 per cent oxygen, which is five per cent less than in the air that we breathe in. By giving rescue breaths, you can force air into the casualty's airway. This air reaches the air sacs (alveoli) in the lungs and oxygen is then transferred to the small blood vessels within the lungs.

Rescue breathing forces air into casualty's lungs

Resuscitation techniques

This section sets out the life-saving measures needed to ensure that an adequate supply of oxygen reaches the vital organs, such as the brain, heart, and kidneys, in an unconscious casualty. It is divided into three main parts: for adults, for children aged one to puberty, and for infants (children under one year old). Each part outlines initial checks, the recovery position, and then describes the techniques – chest compressions and rescue breathing (cardiopulmonary resuscitation or CPR) – that you need to help restore and maintain a casualty's breathing and circulation.

Resuscitation plan

This plan is a summary of all the different stages that are needed to resuscitate an unconscious adult, child, or infant. You can perform all the various stages of resuscitation kneeling next to the casualty's head or chest.

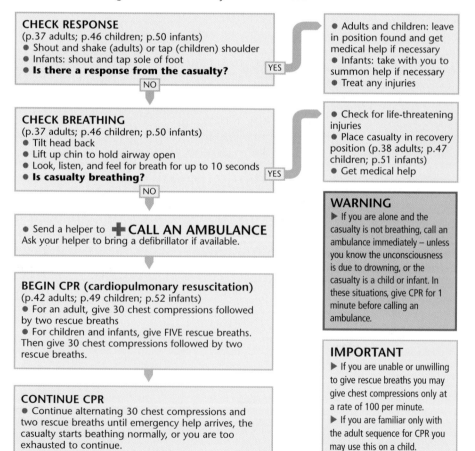

CHECK RESPONSE
(p.37 adults; p.46 children; p.50 infants)
- Shout and shake (adults) or tap (children) shoulder
- Infants: shout and tap sole of foot
- **Is there a response from the casualty?** `YES`

- Adults and children: leave in position found and get medical help if necessary
- Infants: take with you to summon help if necessary
- Treat any injuries

`NO`

CHECK BREATHING
(p.37 adults; p.46 children; p.50 infants)
- Tilt head back
- Lift up chin to hold airway open
- Look, listen, and feel for breath for up to 10 seconds
- **Is casualty breathing?** `YES`

- Check for life-threatening injuries
- Place casualty in recovery position (p.38 adults; p.47 children; p.51 infants)
- Get medical help

`NO`

- Send a helper to ✚ **CALL AN AMBULANCE**
Ask your helper to bring a defibrillator if available.

BEGIN CPR (cardiopulmonary resuscitation)
(p.42 adults; p.49 children; p.52 infants)
- For an adult, give 30 chest compressions followed by two rescue breaths
- For children and infants, give FIVE rescue breaths. Then give 30 chest compressions followed by two rescue breaths.

CONTINUE CPR
- Continue alternating 30 chest compressions and two rescue breaths until emergency help arrives, the casualty starts beathing normally, or you are too exhausted to continue.

WARNING
▶ If you are alone and the casualty is not breathing, call an ambulance immediately – unless you know the unconsciousness is due to drowning, or the casualty is a child or infant. In these situations, give CPR for 1 minute before calling an ambulance.

IMPORTANT
▶ If you are unable or unwilling to give rescue breaths you may give chest compressions only at a rate of 100 per minute.
▶ If you are familiar only with the adult sequence for CPR you may use this on a child.

ADULT LIFE-SAVING SEQUENCE

Check response

▼

If casualty does not respond, **check breathing**

▼

If casualty is breathing normally, place in recovery position

OR

If casualty is not breathing, or has agonal breathing

▼

➕ CALL AN AMBULANCE

▼

Begin chest compressions

▼

Begin rescue breaths

▼

Continue chest compressions and rescue breaths (CPR)

Check response (adult)

If you discover a collapsed casualty, you need to decide if he is conscious or unconscious. Follow the instructions below for an adult casualty.

Check consciousness

- Gently shake the casualty's shoulders and ask "What has happened?" or give a command such as "Open your eyes".

If the casualty responds,
- leave her in the position in which you found her and get help if necessary. Treat any injuries.

If the casualty does not respond,
- shout for help. If you can, leave her in the position in which you found her and open the airway and check breathing (below).

Check breathing (adult)

If the casualty is unconscious, you should open her airway and check breathing.

1 Open airway

- Place one hand on the casualty's forehead and gently tilt her head back.
- Lift the chin with the index and middle fingers of your other hand.

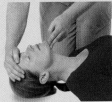

2 Look, listen, and feel for breathing

- Look along the chest for movement, listen for breathing, and feel for breath on your cheek for 10 seconds.

If the casualty is breathing,
- check for life-threatening injuries.
- place her in the recovery position (overleaf).

If the casualty is not breathing or has agonal breathing,
- send a helper, if available, to
➕ CALL AN AMBULANCE
- start chest compressions (p.40).

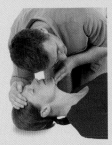

ADULT LIFE-SAVING SEQUENCE

Check response

⬇

If casualty does not respond, check breathing

⬇

If casualty is breathing normally, place in **recovery position**

OR

If casualty is not breathing, or has agonal breathing

⬇

✚ **CALL AN AMBULANCE**

⬇

Begin chest compressions

⬇

Begin rescue breaths

⬇

Continue chest compressions and rescue breaths (CPR)

Recovery position (adult)

If the casualty is unconscious but breathing normally, place her in the recovery position. Follow the instructions below if she is lying on her back. If she is already lying on her side, do not follow entire sequence, but make sure she is in a stable position and cannot roll onto her back.

1 Remove spectacles and bulky objects from pockets

● Straighten the casualty's legs.
● Remove spectacles, if she is wearing them, and any bulky items, such as a mobile phone, from her pockets.

2 Move arm nearest to you

● Place the arm nearest to you at a right angle to the casualty's body, with the palm facing up.

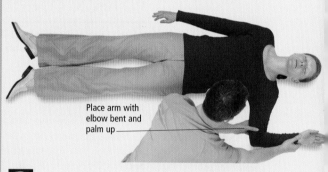

Place arm with elbow bent and palm up

3 Move other arm and raise leg

● Bring the arm furthest from you across the casualty's chest and hold her hand, palm outwards, against the cheek nearest to you.
● With your other hand, get hold of the knee furthest from you and pull the leg up until the foot is flat on the floor.

Pull casualty's knee up

4 Pull knee towards you

- With one hand, keep the casualty's hand pressed against her cheek to support the head.
- With your other hand, pull the leg towards you, rolling the casualty onto her side.

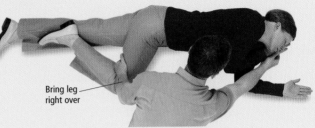

Bring leg right over

5 Position leg at right angle

- Pull the casualty's top leg up at a right angle to the body, so that both the hip and knee are bent at right angles.

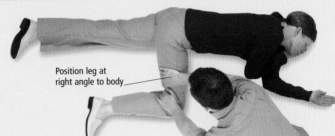

Position leg at right angle to body

6 Keep airway open

- Make sure the casualty's airway remains open.
- If the hand under her cheek has moved, put it back into position to help keep the head tilted.

✚ CALL AN AMBULANCE

7 Monitor casualty

- Monitor and record the casualty's vital signs – level of response, pulse, and breathing (pp.20–1) – regularly until help arrives.

For a suspected spinal injury

If you suspect a casualty has a spinal injury, place her in the recovery position if you are unable to keep her airway open using the jaw-thrust method (p.111) or if you are alone and have to leave her to get help. It is important to keep her neck and back as straight as you can while putting her in the recovery position. This is easier to do if you have one or more helpers.

- If there is no-one to help you, follow the instructions given on these two pages.
- If there is one helper, one person holds the head steady as the other turns the casualty.
- If there are two helpers available, one person holds the casualty's head steady, one turns her, the third keeps the casualty's back straight while she is being turned.

ADULT LIFE-SAVING SEQUENCE

Check response

⬇

If casualty does not respond, check breathing

⬇

If casualty is breathing normally, place in recovery position

OR

If casualty is not breathing, or has agonal breathing

⬇

✚ CALL AN AMBULANCE

⬇

Begin **chest compressions**

⬇

Begin rescue breaths

⬇

Continue chest compressions and rescue breaths (CPR)

Chest compressions (adult)

If the casualty is not breathing, or has agonal breathing (p.35), you should begin cardiopulmonary resuscitation (CPR), which is a combination of chest compressions (below) and rescue breaths (p.42), to simulate blood circulation and breathing. For CPR for children, see page 49; for infants, see page 52.

1 Place hand on centre of chest

● Place the heel of one hand on the centre of the casualty's chest. This is the point where you will apply pressure. You can do this through clothing.

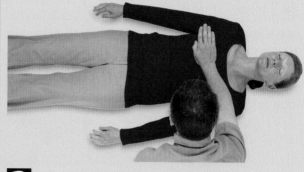

2 Cover hand

● Cover the first hand with your other hand and interlock your fingers.
● Make sure the fingers of both hands underneath are lifted clear of the casualty's chest.
● Make sure you do not press on the ribs, the bottom tip of the breastbone, or the soft upper abdomen.

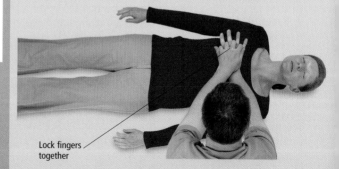

Lock fingers together

3 Give chest compressions

- Kneel up with your shoulders over the breastbone and your arms straight.
- Press down 4–5 cm (1½–2 in).
- Release the pressure on the chest to let it come back up, but do not remove your hands.
- Give 30 chest compressions in total at a rate of 100 per minute.

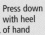
Press down with heel of hand

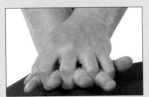
Detail of hands on chest

4 Give rescue breaths

- After you have given 30 chest compressions, give two rescue breaths (overleaf).

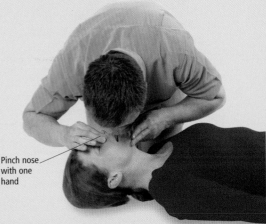
Pinch nose with one hand

IMPORTANT

▶ Continue cycles of 30 compressions to two rescue breaths until medical help arrives and takes over, the casualty starts breathing normally or you become too exhausted to continue.

▶ If you have a helper, swap over every two minutes (after a set of 30 compressions) with as little disruption as possible. This is to maintain good quality of compressions.

ADULT LIFE-SAVING SEQUENCE

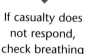

Check response

⬇

If casualty does not respond, check breathing

⬇

If casualty is breathing normally, place in recovery position

OR

If casualty is not breathing, or has agonal breathing

⬇

✚ CALL AN AMBULANCE

⬇

Begin chest compressions

⬇

Begin **rescue breaths**

⬇

Continue chest compressions and rescue breaths (CPR)

Rescue breathing (adult)

If an adult casualty is not breathing normally, you will need to follow chest compressions with rescue breaths.

1 Keep airway open

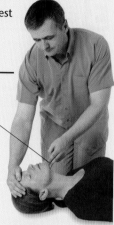

- Make sure the casualty's head remains tilted back by keeping one hand on her forehead and supporting her chin with the index and middle fingers of your other hand.

Support chin

2 Begin rescue breaths

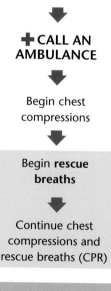

- Pinch the casualty's nose.
- Take a deep breath, and then seal your lips over the casualty's mouth.
- Blow firmly and steadily into the mouth for about 1 second, and watch the chest rise.
- If you cannot blow into her mouth, close it and seal your lips around her nose. After each breath open her mouth to allow the air to escape from the lungs.

Pinch nose with one hand

Using a face shield

A plastic face shield (p.23) reduces the risk of infection when giving rescue breaths.
- Place the face shield over the casualty's face with the filter over the mouth.
- Pinch his nose and give rescue breaths through the filter.

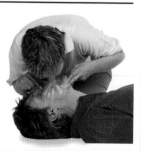

3 Repeat breath

- Lift your mouth away from the casualty's mouth and look at her chest. If the chest rises as you blow and falls when you remove your mouth, you have given a rescue breath.
- Give a second rescue breath.
- If the chest does not rise, check that her head is far enough back and that you have closed her nose completely. Check the mouth and remove any obvious obstruction.
- Make no more than two attempts at rescue breaths before returning to chest compressions.

Watch chest fall

4 Repeat chest compressions

- Give another 30 chest compressions.
- Continue alternating 30 chest compressions with two rescue breaths until the emergency services arrive, the casualty starts breathing normally, or you are too exhausted to continue.

IMPORTANT

▶ If you have a helper, swap over every two minutes (after a set of 30 compressions) with as little disruption as possible. This is to maintain good quality of compressions.

5 Put in recovery position

- If the casualty begins to breathe normally, place her in the recovery position (p.38).
- Monitor and record her vital signs (pp.20–1) regularly until help arrives.

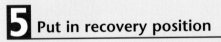

Using a defibrillator

When a casualty has a cardiac arrest, the heart stops beating so there is no circulation. A cardiac arrest may occur after a heart attack in which the normal heart rhythm is disturbed, causing a condition known as ventricular fibrillation. A machine known as an automated external defibrillator (AED), or defibrillator, can be used to try to reverse abnormal heart rhythm and restart a heart. Defibrillators can be found in many public places, including airports, railway stations, shopping centres, and offices, where staff are trained in their use. To use a defibrillator you must be properly trained and able to carry out cardiopulmonary resuscitation (CPR). In most cases when a defibrillator is called for, you will have already started CPR, continue CPR while the defibrillator is prepared, then follow the prompts from the machine.

1 Get defibrillator ready

● Switch on the defibrillator and take out the pads.

2 Remove casualty's upper clothing

● Remove or cut through any clothing covering the chest and wipe away any sweat with a dry cloth.
● Shave the chest hair only if there is so much of it that it will stop the pads sticking to the skin.

3 Put pads on chest

● Attach the pads. Place one pad on the upper right side of the casualty's chest, place the other one on the left side of the chest positioned so that its long axis is vertical.
● Stand clear and make sure no one is touching the casualty because this will prevent the machine from making an accurate analysis.

WARNING
▶ If at any time the casualty starts breathing normally, place him in the recovery position (p.38), leaving the defibrillator attached.
▶ Do not use a defibrillator on a child under the age of one year.

4 Follow defibrillator prompts

● Follow the spoken or visual prompts given by the machine. It will tell you when to give a shock, and when to do CPR. If you need to give a shock, make sure no-one is touching the casualty.
● Continue to follow the prompts until the emergency services arrive and take over from you.
● Do not remove the pads or switch off the defibrillator, even if the casualty appears to have recovered.

Make sure helper does not touch casualty while machine is analysing or delivering a shock

Follow spoken or visual prompts of defibrillator

Position pads either side of heart

Sequence for using a defibrillator

When you use a defibrillator, it will give you a series of spoken and visual prompts (these vary from one machine to another). Once the pads are attached to a casualty's chest, the defibrillator will analyse his heart rhythm and advise you whether or not to give a shock. The chart below outlines the sequence for using the machine and what you should do.

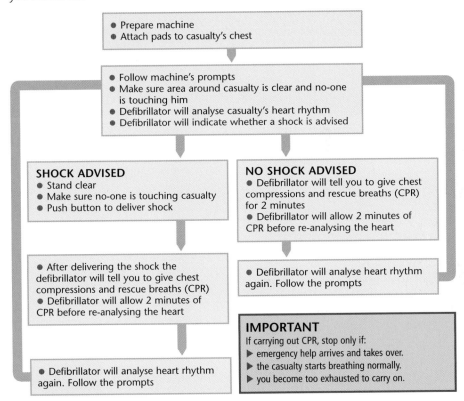

- Prepare machine
- Attach pads to casualty's chest

- Follow machine's prompts
- Make sure area around casualty is clear and no-one is touching him
- Defibrillator will analyse casualty's heart rhythm
- Defibrillator will indicate whether a shock is advised

SHOCK ADVISED
- Stand clear
- Make sure no-one is touching casualty
- Push button to deliver shock

NO SHOCK ADVISED
- Defibrillator will tell you to give chest compressions and rescue breaths (CPR) for 2 minutes
- Defibrillator will allow 2 minutes of CPR before re-analysing the heart

- After delivering the shock the defibrillator will tell you to give chest compressions and rescue breaths (CPR)
- Defibrillator will allow 2 minutes of CPR before re-analysing the heart

- Defibrillator will analyse heart rhythm again. Follow the prompts

IMPORTANT
If carrying out CPR, stop only if:
▶ emergency help arrives and takes over.
▶ the casualty starts breathing normally.
▶ you become too exhausted to carry on.

- Defibrillator will analyse heart rhythm again. Follow the prompts

Paediatric defibrillators

Standard defibrillators can be used for children over the age of eight years. Paediatric defibrillators, or paediatric pads and a standard machine should be used on children aged one to seven years if possible. If neither is available, then use a standard machine. Do not use a defibrillator on a child aged under one year.

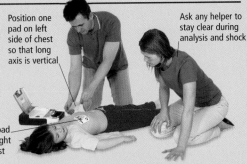

Position one pad on left side of chest so that long axis is vertical

Ask any helper to stay clear during analysis and shock

Place one pad on upper right side of chest

CHILD LIFE-SAVING SEQUENCE

Check response

⬇

If child does not respond, **check breathing**

⬇

If child is breathing, place in **recovery position**

OR

If child is not breathing,

⬇

Ask a helper to ✚ **CALL AN AMBULANCE**

⬇

Give five rescue breaths

⬇

Begin chest compressions with rescue breaths (CPR)

⬇

Repeat for 1 minute and ✚ **CALL AN AMBULANCE** if one has not already been called

⬇

Continue CPR

Check response (child)

If a child has collapsed, you need to find out if he is conscious and breathing. Follow the instructions below for a child aged one to puberty. See page 50 for an infant.

Check consciousness

● Call out the child's name, or give a command such as "Open your eyes", to try to provoke a response.

WARNING
▶ Never shake a child to check if he is conscious or not.

● Tap him on the shoulder.
If the child responds,
● leave him in the position in which you found him and get help if necessary. Treat any injuries.
If the child does not respond,
● shout for help.
● Open the airway and check breathing (below).

Check breathing (child)

If the child is unconscious, open her airway, and check to see if he is breathing normally.

1 Open airway

● Place one hand on the child's forehead and gently tilt the head back.
● Lift the chin with the index and middle fingers of your other hand.
● Do not push on the soft part of the chin as it can block the airway.

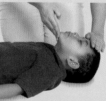

2 Look, listen, and feel for breathing

● Look along the chest for movement, listen for breathing, and feel for breath on your cheek for 10 seconds.
If the child is breathing normally,
● check for life-threatening injuries.
● place him in the recovery position (opposite).
If the child is not breathing,
● send a helper to
✚ **CALL AN AMBULANCE**
● begin rescue breathing (p.48).

Recovery position (child)

If a child aged between one year and puberty is unconscious and breathing, you should place her in the recovery position. If she is already lying on her side, you should make sure that she cannot roll onto her back as this may affect her breathing.

1 Straighten legs and position arm

- Kneel beside the child.
- Straighten her legs.
- Remove spectacles and any bulky items from the pockets.
- Place the arm closest to you at a right angle to the child's body.

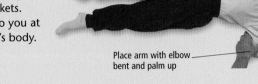

Place arm with elbow bent and palm up

2 Move other arm and raise leg

- Bring the child's far arm across her chest.
- Hold her hand, palm outwards, against her near cheek.
- With your other hand, grasp the knee furthest from you and pull the leg up until the foot is flat on the floor.

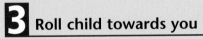

Place foot flat on ground

3 Roll child towards you

- With one hand, keep the child's hand pressed against her cheek to support her head.
- With the other hand, pull her far leg towards you, rolling her onto her side.
- Adjust the upper leg so that both the hip and the knee are bent at right angles.
- Tilt her head back to make sure her airway remains open.

✚ CALL AN AMBULANCE

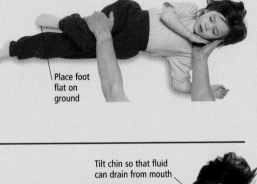

Tilt chin so that fluid can drain from mouth

Pull bent leg towards you

4 Monitor child

- Monitor and record the child's vital signs – level of response, pulse, and breathing (pp.20–1) – regularly until help arrives.

IMPORTANT
▶ If you think that the child might have damaged her neck or spine, follow the instructions given on page 39 for placing someone with a suspected spinal injury into the recovery position.

CHILD LIFE-SAVING SEQUENCE

Check response

⬇

If child does not respond, check breathing

⬇

If child is breathing, place in recovery position

OR

If child is not breathing,

⬇

Ask a helper to
✚ **CALL AN AMBULANCE**

⬇

Give five **rescue breaths**

⬇

Begin **chest compressions** with rescue breaths (CPR)

⬇

Repeat for 1 minute and
✚ **CALL AN AMBULANCE**
if one has not already been called

⬇

Continue CPR

Rescue breathing (child)

If a child aged between one year and puberty is not breathing normally, you will need to give rescue breaths.

1 Keep airway open

● Make sure the child's head is tilted back by keeping one hand on his forehead and his chin is lifted by placing the index and middle fingers of your other hand on the point of his chin.

2 Clear any obstructions from mouth

● Look in the child's mouth for obvious obstructions.
● Pick out anything you see with your thumb and forefinger.
● Do not do a fingersweep of his mouth.

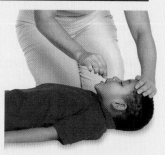

3 Give rescue breaths

● Pinch the child's nose. Take a deep breath, open your mouth, and seal your lips over the child's mouth.
● Blow firmly and steadily into the mouth for about about 1 second, watch the chest rise.
● Give FIVE rescue breaths.
● If the chest does not rise, check that his head is far enough back and that you have closed his nose completely.
● After five breaths (or attempts at breaths) begin chest compressions, opposite.

Blow into child's mouth to give rescue breaths

Chest compressions (child)

If a child is not breathing normally, start CPR – a combination of chest compressions (below) and rescue breaths (opposite). If you are alone, do 1 minute of CPR before you call an ambulance.

1 Position hand on chest

- Place the heel of one hand on the centre of the child's chest. This is the point at which you press down on the chest to give chest compressions.
- Take care not to press on the ribs, the lower tip of the breastbone, or the soft upper abdomen.

Press down straight with heel of hand, keeping fingers lifted

2 Give chest compressions

- Lean over the child, keeping your arm straight and keep your fingers lifted so you do not press down onto the ribs.
- Press down vertically on the breastbone with the heel of your hand to one third of the depth of the child's chest.
- Release the pressure on the chest to let it come back up, but do not remove your hands. Let the chest come back up.
- Do this 30 times at a rate of 100 compressions per minute.

IMPORTANT
▶ If the child starts breathing normally, place him in the recovery position (p.47).

3 Give two rescue breaths

- After giving 30 chest compressions, tilt the child's head back, lift the chin, and give TWO rescue breaths (opposite).

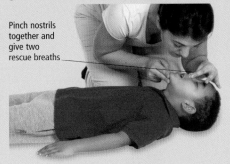

Pinch nostrils together and give two rescue breaths

4 Alternate compressions with rescue breaths

- Carry on giving cycles of 30 chest compressions and two rescue breaths, maintaining the rate of 100 compressions per minute, for 1 minute.

✚ **CALL AN AMBULANCE**

- Continue until help arrives and takes over, the child starts breathing, or you become too exhausted to continue.

For a larger child or small first aider

If you are small, or the child is large, give compressions with two hands as for an adult.

- Place one hand on the centre of the child's chest.
- Cover with your other hand and interlock your fingers, keeping your fingers raised.

INFANT LIFE-SAVING SEQUENCE

Check response

If infant does
not respond,
check breathing

If infant is
breathing, place in
recovery position

OR

If infant is not
breathing,

Ask a helper to
➕ **CALL AN
AMBULANCE**

Give five **rescue breaths**

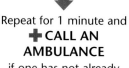

Begin chest
compressions with
rescue breaths (CPR)

Repeat for 1 minute and
➕ **CALL AN
AMBULANCE**
if one has not already
been called

Continue CPR

Check response (infant)

This sequence is for an infant under the age of one year. It is easier to treat an infant if you place him on his back on a firm, flat surface at about waist height.

Check consciousness

● Tap the sole of the infant's foot and call his name, if you know it.

If the infant responds,
● take him with you to get medical help if needed. Treat any injuries.

If the infant does not respond,
● shout for help.
● Open the airway and check breathing (below).

> **WARNING**
> ▶ Never shake an infant to check if he is conscious.

Check breathing (infant)

If the infant is unconscious, open his airway and check to see if he is breathing normally.

1 Open airway

● Place one hand on the infant's forehead and gently tilt the head back.
● Lift the infant's chin using one finger of your other hand.
● Do not push on the soft part of the chin as it can block the airway.

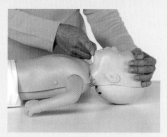

2 Look, listen, and feel for breathing

● Look along the chest for movement, listen for breathing, and feel for breath on your cheek for 10 seconds.

If the infant is breathing normally,
● check for life-threatening injuries.
● hold him in the recovery position (opposite).

If the infant is not breathing,
● send a helper to
➕ **CALL AN AMBULANCE**
● begin rescue breathing (opposite).

Recovery position (infant)

If an unconscious infant is breathing normally, hold him in the recovery position with his head lower than his body. This will keep his airway open, allow any vomit or fluids to drain from his mouth, and keep his neck and spine aligned and stable.

1 Keep airway open

- Cradle the infant in your arms with his head lower than his body, to prevent him from choking on his tongue or inhaling his vomit.
- ✚ **CALL AN AMBULANCE**

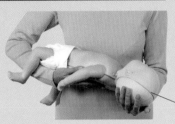

Head is lower than body

2 Monitor infant

- Monitor and record the infant's vital signs – level of response, pulse, and breathing (pp.20–1) – regularly until help arrives.

Rescue breathing (infant)

If an unconscious infant is not breathing normally, you will need to begin rescue breaths to get oxygen into the lungs.

1 Keep airway open

- Make sure the infant's head is tilted back and the chin is lifted.

2 Clear any obstructions

- Pick out any obvious obstructions from the mouth with your finger and thumb.
- Do not do a fingersweep of the mouth.

3 Give rescue breaths

- Take a breath and place your lips around the infant's mouth and nose to form an airtight seal.
- Blow firmly and steadily for about 1second, until you see the chest rise.
- Lift your mouth away from the infant's face and see if his chest falls.
- Give five rescue breaths.

- If the chest does not rise, check that his head is far enough back and that you have an effective seal around the infant's mouth and nose.

4 Begin chest compressions

- After five breaths (or attempts at breaths) begin chest compressions (p.52).

Pick out visible obstructions

Maintain an airtight seal

INFANT LIFE-SAVING SEQUENCE

Check response

⬇

If infant does not respond, check breathing

⬇

If infant is breathing, place in recovery position

OR

If infant is not breathing,

⬇

Ask a helper to
✚ **CALL AN AMBULANCE**

⬇

Give five rescue breaths

⬇

Begin **chest compressions** with rescue breaths (CPR)

⬇

Repeat for 1 minute and
✚ **CALL AN AMBULANCE**
if one has not already been called

⬇

Continue CPR

Chest compressions
(infant)

If a infant is not breathing normally, start CPR – a combination of chest compressions (below) and rescue breaths (opposite). If you are alone, do 1 minute of CPR before you call an ambulance.

1 Give chest compressions

● Lay the infant on a firm, flat surface, either at roughly waist height or on the floor.
● Place the fingertips of your index and middle fingers on the centre of his chest.
● Press down one third of the depth of the infant's chest. Release the pressure on the chest without losing the contact between your fingers and the breastbone. Let the chest come back up.
● Press down on the chest 30 times in total at a rate of 100 times per minute.

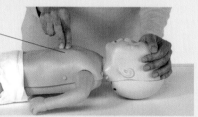

Press down to one third of depth of infant's chest

2 Give rescue breaths

● After you have given 30 chest compressions, tilt the infant's head, lift the chin, and give two more rescue breaths through the mouth and nose (p.51).

3 Alternate chest compressions with rescue breaths

● Continue the cycle of 30 compressions and two rescue breaths until emergency help arrives and takes over, the infant starts breathing normally, or you become so exhausted that you cannot carry on.

IMPORTANT
▶ If you are alone and the infant is not breathing, complete 1 minute of CPR before taking the infant with you to call an ambulance.

Choking (adult)

An object such as a piece of food stuck at the back of the throat can block the windpipe and result in choking. If the blockage remains, the casualty may lose consciousness, so prompt first aid is vital. Follow the steps below for adults, and children over puberty; see page 54 for younger children, and page 55 for infants.

Your aims
▶ Clear obstruction from throat
▶ Get casualty to hospital if necessary

SIGNS AND SYMPTOMS
▶ With mild choking: red face and coughing
▶ With severe obstruction: unable to speak, cough, or breathe

---

1 Give casualty back blows

● If choking is mild and he is coughing, encourage him to continue.
● If obstruction is severe and he stops breathing, bend him forwards. Stand behind him and give a sharp blow between his shoulderblades. Repeat back blows up to five times.
● Check the mouth to see if the object has been dislodged. Remove the object.

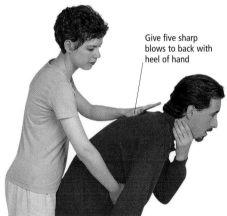

Give five sharp blows to back with heel of hand

2 Prepare for abdominal thrusts

● If the back blows fail, stand behind the casualty and place a clenched fist with thumb side in over his upper abdomen just below the ribs.

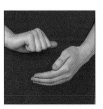

3 Give abdominal thrusts

● Grasp your fist and pull inwards and upwards, up to five times.
● Check the mouth to see if the object has been dislodged. Remove the object.

Pull inwards and upwards

4 Repeat steps 1 to 3

● If he is still choking after three cycles of back blows and abdominal thrusts,
✚ **CALL AN AMBULANCE**
● Continue to alternate back blows and abdominal thrusts until help arrives.

WARNING
▶ If the casualty loses consciousness, open the airway, check breathing, and give chest compressions (p.42) to try to dislodge the object.
✚ **CALL AN AMBULANCE**
▶ If given abdominal thrusts he must see a doctor.

Choking (child)

Young children can easily choke on food or small objects. Your priority is to remove the obstruction and clear the airway as quickly as possible. Follow the instructions below for children between the age of one year and puberty.

Your aims
▶ Clear obstruction from throat
▶ Get child to hospital if necessary

SIGNS AND SYMPTOMS
▶ With mild choking: red face, and coughing
▶ With severe obstruction: inability to speak, cough, or breathe

1 Give back blows

● If the choking is mild and the child is coughing, encourage him to continue.
● If obstruction is severe and he stops coughing or breathing, bend him forwards.
● Stand or kneel behind him and give a sharp blow between the shoulderblades with the heel of your hand (back blow). Repeat up to five times.
● Check the child's mouth and pick out any visible obstructions.

Bend child forwards

2 Give abdominal thrusts

● If back blows fail, hold one fist against the abdomen. Grasp your fist with your other hand and pull inwards and upwards. Do this up to five times.
● Check the mouth and pick out any obstructions.

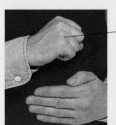

Place fist with thumb against abdomen

Give five abdominal thrusts

WARNING
▶ If the child loses consciousness, open the airway, check breathing, and if not breathing, give five rescue breaths (pp.46, 48). Then give chest compressions (p.49) to try to dislodge the object, followed by rescue breaths.

✚ **CALL AN AMBULANCE**

▶ If a child is given abdominal thrusts he must be seen by a doctor.

3 Repeat steps 1 and 2

● If the child is still choking after three cycles of steps 1 and 2,
✚ **CALL AN AMBULANCE**
● Repeat steps 1 and 2 until help arrives.

Choking (infant)

If an infant's airway is partially blocked, he may be distressed and coughing. If it is completely blocked, he will be unable to breathe or cough and will quickly become unconscious. For a choking infant, follow the instructions below.

Your aims
▶ Clear obstruction from throat
▶ Get infant to hospital if necessary

SIGNS AND SYMPTOMS
▶ With mild choking: infant has red face, is able to cry, and cough
▶ With severe obstruction: infant has difficulty crying, or making any noise, and unable to breathe

1 Give infant back blows

● If the infant is unable to cough or cry, lay face down along your forearm.
● Give infant up to five sharp back blows with the heel of your hand.

Give back blows with heel of your hand

3 Give chest thrusts

● Lay the infant face up on your arm.
● Give up to five downward thrusts to the chest.
● Check the mouth for any obstructions and pick them out.

Use two fingers to give chest thrusts

2 Pick out any obstructions

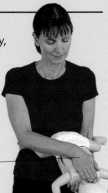

● Check the infant's mouth.
● Remove any visible obstructions using your fingertips.

Look for obstructions in mouth

4 Repeat steps 1 to 3

● If the obstruction has still not cleared after three cycles of steps 1–3, keep the infant with you and
✚ CALL AN AMBULANCE
● Repeat steps 1–3 until help arrives.

WARNING
▶ If the infant loses consciousness, open the airway, check breathing, and if not breathing, give five rescue breaths (pp.50–1). Then begin chest compressions (p.52) to try to dislodge the object, followed by rescue breaths.
✚ CALL AN AMBULANCE

IMPORTANT
▶ Do not put your fingers down the infant's throat to feel for, or attempt to remove, an obstruction.
▶ Do not use abdominal thrusts on an infant.

Test yourself

Now that you have read and studied the chapter on life-saving techniques, see if you can answer the questions below. After completing the questions, check your answers against the correct ones on page 144.

1 What does ABC stand for in the ABC of resuscitation?

A...
B...
C ....

2 Which organ pumps blood around the body?

....
....

3 What is the correct order for treating an unconscious casualty?

Put him in recovery position ....
Open airway ....
Call ambulance ....
Check breathing ....

4 How long should it take to give a rescue breath?

One second ....
Two seconds ....
Three seconds ....

5 When and why is it good practice to use a face shield?

....
....
....
....
....
....
....
....
....
....

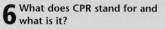

6 What does CPR stand for and what is it?

....
....
....
....
....

7 Which is the correct place to press down when giving chest compressions?

a Upper half of the chest...................☐
b Lower half of the chest...................☐
c Centre of the chest ....☐

8 When starting CPR, how many chest compressions and rescue breaths should you give and in what order. At what rate should you give the chest compressions? Answer for an adult, child, and infant casualty.

Adult...
....
....
Child...
....
Infant...
....
....

9 What is a defibrillator?

....
....
....

10 Which of the following indicate that a casualty could be choking?

a Red face.....................................☐
b Swollen hands..............................☐
c Clutching the throat ....☐
d Coughing....................................☐
e Rapid breathing through the mouth....................................☐
f Difficulty breathing ....☐

11 Which of the following techniques should not be used on a conscious infant who is choking?

Chest thrusts...
Back blows..
Abdominal thrusts ....

3 Wounds and bleeding

A wound is a break in the body's protective layer – the skin. This break allows germs to enter the body, causing possible infection and blood to escape. Severe blood loss is serious because oxygen is carried around the body by blood. If too much blood is lost, then insufficient oxygen is supplied to the tissues, resulting in a potentially life-threatening medical condition called shock.

Clear anatomical information explains what happens when blood vessels are damaged to help you understand why first-aid treatments are effective. This chapter clearly sets out general principles that apply to treating any wounds and bleeding. There are guidelines, too, for adapting the techniques when necessary for minor cuts and grazes or serious wounds such as amputation.

Use the questionnaire on page 74 to test your understanding of the procedures described in this chapter.

Contents

Dealing with severe bleeding	58
Blood vessels and bleeding	60
Shock	61
Cuts and grazes	62
Bruising	63
Blisters	63
Crush injury	64
Amputation	65
Eye wound	66
Scalp wound	66
Nosebleed	67
Ear wound	67
Mouth wound	68
Knocked-out tooth	68
Wound to palm	69
Embedded object	70
Splinters	72
Fish-hook injury	73
Test yourself	74

Dealing with severe bleeding

Blood loss can be serious and should be controlled as soon as possible. If the casualty loses a lot of blood, a condition called shock will develop, and eventually he will lose consciousness. If the bleeding is external, there will be a wound visible in the skin from which blood is escaping. Only approach the casualty if it is safe to do so. Assess the wound, check for embedded objects, and ask the casualty what has happened. Severe bleeding can be distressing, so explain what you are doing to reassure him. Make sure you avoid pressing on any foreign object in the wound.

Recognising shock
Look for signs of shock, such as pallor and sweating. The casualty may complain of nausea, faintness, and dizziness

Apply pressure
Using either your hand or the casualty's hand, apply pressure directly onto the wound. If there is an embedded object in the wound, press on either side of it

Elevate limb
Raise wound above the level of the heart, if possible, to reduce bleeding

Check for bleeding
Look for evidence of severe external blood loss on the casualty's clothes

Make casualty comfortable
Encourage casualty to sit down in a comfortable position

Get a history
Ask the casualty how the injury occurred

Check for danger
Make sure that the cause of injury does not pose any further threat and that there are no additional risks to you or the casualty

What you should do

Your aims
▶ Control bleeding
▶ Prevent infection
▶ Prevent shock if possible
▶ Get casualty to hospital urgently

IMPORTANT
▶ Take care with hygiene – wear disposable gloves if available.
▶ Do not allow the casualty to eat, drink, or smoke in case a general anaesthetic is needed in hospital.

1 Examine wound

● Check the wound to make sure there are no embedded objects (p.70).

2 Apply pressure to wound

● Press on the wound with your fingers or palm, ideally over a sterile dressing or clean pad. You can ask the casualty to do this while you put on disposable gloves.
● If there is an embedded object, press on either side of the object.

3 Raise and support limb

● If the casualty is bleeding from a limb, raise and support the limb above the level of his heart.

4 Dress wound

● Secure the dressing over the wound with a roller bandage.
● If blood seeps through, put on a second dressing.
● If blood seeps through the second dressing, remove both dressings and start again, making sure pressure is accurately applied over the wound.

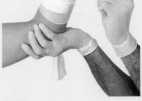

Maintain pressure with bandage

5 Check for shock

● Help the casualty to lie down and watch for signs of shock (p.61).
● Phone for an ambulance.
● Monitor and record the casualty's vital signs – level of response, pulse, and breathing (pp.20–1) – regularly until help arrives.

Blood vessels and bleeding

In the body of the average adult, there are about 6 litres (10 ½ pints) of blood, or about 1 litre (1¾ pints) of blood per 13kg (28lbs) of body weight, circulating around the body. The main component of blood is a fluid called plasma. This fluid contains red and white blood cells and also platelets, which help the blood to clot. Blood is carried around the body by vessels called arteries, capillaries, and veins (right). If blood vessels are damaged, they constrict at the site of the injury and the blood-clotting process begins (below).

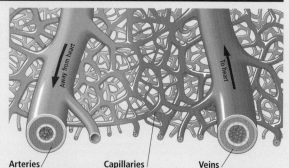

Arteries
These blood vessels have muscular walls through which blood travels at high pressure. Arteries carry blood containing oxygen from the heart to the tissues.

Capillaries
These tiny, thin-walled vessels connect arteries and veins. Their thin walls allow oxygen and nutrients to pass to the body tissues, and waste products such as carbon dioxide to be carried away.

Veins
Blood without oxygen is carried back to the heart through the veins, which have thinner, less muscular walls than arteries.

How blood clots

A blood clot is the solidification of blood that occurs either spontaneously within a blood vessel or as the result of a leakage from the vessel. A clot that forms outside a blood vessel usually occurs in response to damage to that vessel. For example, at the site of a wound, blood leaks from the skin because the blood vessels beneath it are damaged and the blood then solidifies to form a clot (below). At the same time, the blood vessels constrict to limit the flow of blood to the wound.

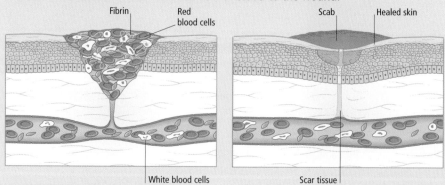

Bleeding from a wound
Small blood cells called platelets clump together at the site of the wound. The platelets and damaged blood vessels then react to form a chemical called thrombin. This, in turn, reacts with a blood protein and creates fibrin filaments to form a mesh at the wound site.

Forming a protective scab
More platelets and red and white blood cells gather together inside the fibrin mesh. The fibrin filaments then contract and a clot is quickly formed. Eventually, the clot hardens and a protective scab forms over the site of the cut, which then heals and may leave a scar.

Shock

This life-threatening condition occurs when the circulation of blood around the body is reduced and vital organs, such as the brain and heart, do not get enough oxygen. Shock is most commonly caused by severe blood loss; it can also be the result of fluid loss due to burns, vomiting, or diarrhoea, or the result of a severe allergic reaction (see Anaphylactic shock p.129). Emergency medical treatment is vital.

<table>
<tr><td>Your aims</td><td>You will need</td></tr>
<tr><td>
▶ Treat obvious causes of shock
▶ Improve circulation
▶ Get casualty to hospital urgently
</td><td>
▶ Blanket/coat
▶ Notepad and pen
</td></tr>
</table>

1 Treat injuries

● Treat any obvious injuries, such as bleeding, burns, or broken bones.

2 Help casualty lie down

● Help the casualty to lie down.
● Raise his legs above the level of his heart if they are not injured.
● Reassure the casualty.

3 Keep casualty warm

● Protect the casualty from extremes of temperature, if necessary by placing a blanket or coat around him.
✚ CALL AN AMBULANCE

4 Monitor casualty

● Monitor and record the casualty's vital signs – level of response, pulse, and breathing (pp.20–1) – regularly until help arrives.

SIGNS AND SYMPTOMS
▶ Pale, cold, and clammy skin
▶ Nausea
▶ Rapid and then weak pulse
▶ Fast and shallow breathing
▶ Restlessness
▶ Yawning and sighing
▶ Thirst
▶ Gradual loss of consciousness; eventual death if treatment is not successful

Internal bleeding

● This can result from damage to an internal organ or from an injury that causes a major bone, such as the pelvis or a thighbone (femur), to break; both of these conditions can cause severe bleeding within the body.
● You should suspect internal bleeding if the casualty is displaying signs of shock, if you notice a large amount of swelling around the site of the injury, or if the casualty is experiencing a marked degree of tenderness around the abdomen.

IMPORTANT
▶ Do not allow the casualty to eat or drink as he may later need a general anaesthetic in hospital.

Monitor and record casualty's vital signs

Cuts and grazes

Small cuts and grazes soon stop bleeding without treatment. However, any break in the skin, even a small one, can allow germs to enter the body. Germs are micro-organisms, such as bacteria, that are carried by flies or by unwashed hands; if they are allowed to settle on an open wound, they can cause infection.

Your aims	You will need
▶ Stop wound from becoming infected ▶ Control any bleeding	▶ Disposable gloves ▶ Sterile gauze swabs or antiseptic wipes ▶ Plaster or sterile wound dressing ▶ Bandage

IMPORTANT
▶ Do not handle the open graze or cut with your fingers while you are treating the casualty.
▶ Do not try to remove anything that is embedded in the wound; treat as described on p.70.
▶ Do not use cotton wool on or near an open wound because fibres may stick to the wound.

1 Rinse wound

● Help the casualty to sit down.
● Put on disposable gloves, if available.
● Raise the injured part.
● Rinse the wound under cold running water to remove any dirt or grit.

Rinse wound to remove any dirt

2 Clean around wound

● Using a fresh swab or wipe for each stroke, clean around the wound, working from the edge of the wound outwards.
● Carefully pick off any loose foreign matter, such as glass, metal, or gravel, from or around the wound.

Gently clean around wound

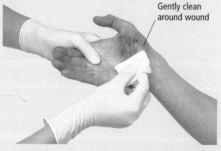

3 Dry around wound

● Without disturbing the wound, gently dry the area around it with a gauze swab.

4 Cover wound

● For a small cut or graze, apply a plaster to the affected area; make sure you do not touch the sterile part of the plaster.
● If the cut or graze is too large for a plaster, cover it with a sterile wound dressing and secure the dressing with the bandage.
● Advise the casualty to rest the injured part and, if possible, to support it in a raised position.

Tetanus immunisation

Tetanus is a serious infection caused by a bacterium that lives in the soil. Infection can be prevented by immunisation. Always ask a casualty with a cut or wound about his tetanus immunisations. Seek medical advice if:
● He has never had a tetanus injection.
● He does not know when he was last injected or how many injections he has had.
● It is more than 10 years since his last tetanus injection.

Bruising

This follows an injury and is caused by bleeding into the skin or into tissues beneath the skin. The area can become blue-black rapidly, or the bruise may take a few days to appear. Bruises that appear quickly will benefit from first aid. Elderly people and those taking blood-thinning (anticoagulant) drugs are likely to bruise particularly easily.

Your aim	You will need
▶ Reduce swelling	▶ Cold compress

1 Support injury

● Support the injured part in the most comfortable position for the casualty.

2 Apply cold compress

● Place a cold compress (p.25) on the bruised area to reduce the blood flow to the injury and relieve pain.
● Press firmly on the compress and keep it in place for at least 5 minutes.

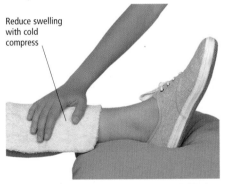

Reduce swelling with cold compress

> **WARNING**
> ▶ A "black eye" is a bruise normally caused by a blow to the face. As it may also cause damage to the eye or skull, you should always seek medical advice.

Blisters

These result from friction or friction burns, which occur when the skin is rubbed repeatedly against a surface. Blisters develop when tissue fluid leaks from the damaged area and collects under the outer layer of the skin.

Your aims	You will need
▶ Relieve pain ▶ Prevent infection	▶ Soap and cold water ▶ Clean pad ▶ Plaster or sterile wound dressing ▶ Adhesive tape/bandage

1 Clean affected area

● Wash the area carefully with soap and cold water and rinse with cold water.

2 Dry affected area

● Using a gentle patting action, dry the area and the surrounding skin very thoroughly with a clean pad.

3 Protect blister

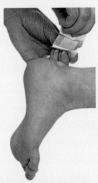

● Carefully cover the blister with a plaster. Make sure the pad of the plaster is larger than the blister.
● If the blister is very large, use a sterile wound dressing or a piece of non-fluffy material, secured with adhesive tape or a bandage.

> **IMPORTANT**
> ▶ Never deliberately burst a blister.

Crush injury

A crush injury is usually the result of a building site incident or a car crash. The injury may include a fracture as well as internal and external bleeding. If a casualty is crushed for a prolonged length of time, body tissues – especially muscles – will be damaged, and when the pressure is released the casualty will go into shock. Toxic chemicals will also build up in the crushed tissues and, if released suddenly into the circulation, they can cause kidney failure. Follow the instructions below if the casualty has been trapped for less than 15 minutes; if the casualty has been trapped for more than 15 minutes, follow the instructions given in the box at the bottom of the page.

Your aims	You will need
▶ Release casualty	▶ Disposable gloves
▶ Treat any injuries	▶ Sterile wound
▶ Get casualty to	dressing/clean pad
hospital urgently	▶ Notepad and pen

1 Remove object

- Put on disposable gloves, if available.
- Remove the object, provided that it has not been there for more than 15 minutes.

Remove object quickly

2 Treat injuries

- Place a sterile wound dressing on any wounds and press firmly to control any bleeding (pp.58–9).
- Immobilise any fractures (pp.102–13).
- Treat the casualty for shock (p.61).

✚ CALL AN AMBULANCE

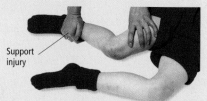

Support injury

3 Monitor casualty

- Monitor and record the casualty's vital signs – level of response, pulse, and breathing (pp.20–1) – regularly until help arrives.

If crushed for more than 15 minutes

IMPORTANT
▶ Do not release the casualty if he has been crushed for more than 15 minutes.

✚ CALL AN AMBULANCE

- Act calmly and reassure the casualty.
- Monitor and record the casualty's vital signs – level of response, pulse, and breathing (pp.20–1) – regularly until help arrives.

Amputation

The complete or partial severing of a limb or digit (finger or toe) is known as amputation. The amputated part can, in many cases, be reattached by microsurgery, so it is important to get the casualty and the severed part to hospital as soon as possible. The casualty is likely to suffer from shock and will need to be treated accordingly.

Your aims	You will need
▶ Minimise blood loss	▶ Disposable gloves
▶ Treat for shock	▶ Sterile wound
▶ Get casualty to	dressing or pad and
hospital urgently	roller bandage
▶ Prevent deterioration	▶ Notepad and pen
of amputated part	For amputated part:
	▶ Kitchen film/
	plastic bag
	▶ Soft fabric
	▶ Ice

2 Secure dressing

● Secure the dressing or pad with a roller bandage (p.26).

✚ CALL AN AMBULANCE

Secure dressing with bandage

1 Control bleeding

● Put on disposable gloves, if available.
● Raise the injured part, then place a sterile wound dressing or clean pad on the wound and press on it firmly to control the bleeding.
● If the digit or limb is partially severed, bring the parts together, wrap the dressing or pad around the wound, and then apply pressure over the wound.
● Make casualty comfortable and treat for shock, if required (p.61).

IMPORTANT
▶ Tell the ambulance service that the casualty has an amputation.
▶ If a digit has been amputated and the casualty is not in shock, you could take him and the amputated part to hospital yourself.

3 Monitor casualty

● Monitor and record his vital signs – level of response, pulse, and breathing (pp.20–1) – regularly until help arrives.

Care of amputated part

● Do not wash the amputated part.
● Wrap the amputated part in kitchen film or put it in a plastic bag.
● Wrap the package in soft fabric and place it in ice, but do not let it come into direct contact with the ice.
● Label the package with the casualty's name and the time of injury.
● Give it to the ambulance personnel.

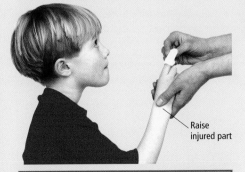

Raise injured part

WARNING
▶ Do not let the casualty eat, drink, or smoke; any microsurgery will require a general anaesthetic.

Eye wound

The eye can be injured by direct blows or by sharp fragments of grit or glass. Even a minor eye injury should be examined promptly by a doctor to prevent any loss of vision. It is important that the casualty remains still during and after treatment.

Your aims	You will need
▶ Cover wounded eye	▶ Disposable gloves
▶ Get casualty to hospital urgently	▶ Gauze pad
	▶ Bandage

SIGNS AND SYMPTOMS
- ▶ Intense pain and fluttering of eyelid
- ▶ Obvious wound to, or bloodshot, eye
- ▶ Problems with vision
- ▶ Leakage of blood or clear fluid from eye

1 Keep casualty still

- Help the casualty to lie on his back, and cradle his head in your lap.
- Tell him not to move his eyes because this may cause further damage.
- Reassure the casualty.

IMPORTANT
- ▶ Do not remove a foreign object in the eye (p.132).
- ▶ For chemical burns to the eye, see p.81.

2 Cover eye

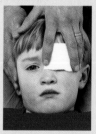

- Put on disposable gloves, if available.
- Cover the injured eye with a gauze pad.

➕ CALL AN AMBULANCE

- If medical help is delayed, secure the dressing in place with a bandage.

Scalp wound

The scalp, the skin covering the head, has many small blood vessels running close to its surface. For this reason, any wound to the scalp can result in profuse bleeding, making an injury appear more serious than it is.

Your aims	You will need
▶ Control bleeding	▶ Disposable gloves
▶ Get casualty to hospital	▶ Sterile wound dressings
	▶ Roller bandage

2 Help casualty lie down

- Help the casualty to lie down with her head and shoulders slightly raised.
- Take or send the casualty to hospital.

1 Control bleeding

- Put on disposable gloves, if available.
- Gently place a sterile wound dressing over the wound.
- Press firmly on the pad.
- Secure the dressing with a roller bandage.
- If blood shows through, secure another sterile dressing on top of the original one.

WARNING
- ▶ If the wound is the result of a blow to the head, treat as for head injury (p.93) and watch for changes to the level of consciousness.

➕ CALL AN AMBULANCE

- ▶ Monitor and record the casualty's vital signs (pp.20–1) regularly until help arrives.

Nosebleed

Bleeding from the nose usually follows a blow to the nose, but it can occur without any apparent cause.

Your aims	You will need
▶ Control bleeding	▶ Tissues
▶ Prevent choking	

1 Ask casualty to sit down

● Ask the casualty to sit down and lean her head forwards.
● Offer her tissues to wipe away blood.
● Loosen her collar if it is tight.

2 Pinch nose

● Tell her to pinch the soft part of her nose for 10 minutes and to breathe through her mouth.
● If the bleeding continues, pinch the nose again.
● While she is pinching her nose, tell her to spit out any blood in her mouth.
● Once bleeding stops, tell the casualty not to blow her nose for several hours, as this may disturb the clot.

IMPORTANT
▶ If the nose is still bleeding after applying pressure for 30 minutes,
➕ **CALL AN AMBULANCE**

WARNING
▶ If yellowish, blood-stained fluid is coming from the nose and/or ear after a blow to the head, it could indicate a skull fracture.
▶ Gently help the casualty to lie down as carefully as possible, and follow the first-aid action as described for head injury (p.93).

Ear wound

The usual cause of a bleeding ear is a burst eardrum, caused by a foreign object or a blow to the head.

Your aims	You will need
▶ Cover wound	▶ Disposable gloves
▶ Get casualty to hospital urgently	▶ Sterile wound dressing

IMPORTANT
▶ Do not attempt to plug the ear.
▶ Do not try to remove a foreign object.

1 Help casualty lie down

● Help the casualty to lie down with his head and shoulders raised.

2 Cover wound

● Put on disposable gloves, if available.
● Place a sterile wound dressing over the ear and lightly secure it with the bandage.
➕ **CALL AN AMBULANCE**

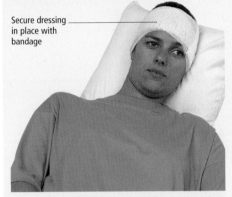

Secure dressing in place with bandage

➕ **CALL AN AMBULANCE**
▶ Monitor and record the casualty's vital signs – level of response, pulse, and breathing (pp.20–1) – regularly until help arrives.

Mouth wound

Cuts to the tongue and lips are usually caused by the casualty's own teeth. Bleeding from the mouth or a tooth socket may also occur straight after losing a tooth or some time after a tooth has been removed by a dentist.

Your aims	You will need
▶ Keep airway clear	▶ Disposable gloves
▶ Control bleeding	▶ Gauze pad

IMPORTANT
▶ Get medical or dental help if the mouth bleeds for longer than 30 minutes, and replace blood-soaked gauze pads with fresh ones.
▶ Tell the casualty not to drink anything hot for 12 hours after the bleeding has stopped.

1 Keep airway clear

● Help the casualty to sit down.
● Lean her forwards and towards the injured side to help the blood drain away and keep the airway clear.

2 Press on wound

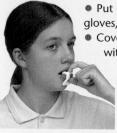

● Put on disposable gloves, if available.
● Cover the wound with a gauze pad.
● Ask the casualty to press the pad onto the wound for 10 minutes.

If a tooth socket is bleeding

● Put a gauze pad over the socket. The pad should be thick enough to stop the top and bottom teeth meeting.
● Tell the casualty to bite on this for 10 minutes.

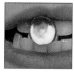

Detail

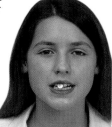

Knocked-out tooth

If an adult tooth has been knocked out, it should be replanted in its socket – the right way round – as soon as possible.

Your aims	You will need
▶ Replant tooth	▶ Disposable gloves
▶ Get casualty to dentist	▶ Gauze pad

1 Replant tooth

● Put on disposable gloves, if available.
● Place tooth back in its socket.
● Place a gauze pad between the top and bottom teeth to keep the tooth in position.
● If the tooth cannot be replanted, tell the casualty to keep the tooth in her cheek or store it in milk or water.

2 Get casualty to dentist

● Take or send the casualty to a dentist.

Carefully put tooth back in socket

Wound to palm

It can be difficult to apply pressure to the wound to control the bleeding with this type of injury. If nothing is embedded in the wound, treat the injury as shown below. If an object is embedded, treat as described on pages 70–1.

Your aims	You will need
▶ Control the bleeding	▶ Disposable gloves
▶ Get casualty to hospital	▶ Sterile wound dressing
	▶ Triangular bandage

1 Apply pressure

● Put on disposable gloves, if available.
● Check the wound to make sure that nothing is embedded in it.
● Apply direct pressure to the wound; either you or the casualty can do this.
● Raise the hand above the level of the heart.

Get casualty to make a fist over pad

Make sure arm is raised and supported

2 Cover wound

● Put a sterile dressing on the wound. Ask the casualty to clench his fist over the pad.
● Roll the bandage around the clenched fist to secure the dressing, leaving the thumb exposed. Tie a reef knot (p.22) over the fingers.

3 Check circulation

● Check the circulation in the thumb on the injured arm (see Roller bandages p.26).
● If the circulation is restricted, loosen the bandage and check the circulation again.

4 Secure arm in sling

● Support the casualty's arm in an elevation sling (p.29).
● Recheck the circulation in the casualty's thumb.

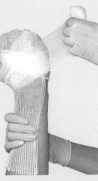

Make sure sling is comfortable

5 Get casualty to hospital

● Take or send the casualty to hospital.

Embedded object

If an object is embedded or stuck in a wound, never try to remove it. The reason is because the object may be plugging the wound, preventing bleeding, and also because you may do more damage by pulling it out. Instead, protect the area with gauze and place a dressing made of spare rolled-up bandages around the object, held in place with another bandage. This will maintain enough pressure to control the bleeding without pressing directly on the wound or the object.

Your aims	You will need
▶ Control bleeding	▶ Disposable gloves
▶ Protect wound from infection	▶ Piece of gauze
▶ Immobilise affected area	▶ Bandages for padding and to cover wound
▶ Get casualty to hospital	

WARNING
▶ If the object is large or embedded near a vital organ or an eye,

✚ **CALL AN AMBULANCE**

1 Control bleeding

- Put on disposable gloves, if available.
- Help the casualty to lie down.
- Pinch the edges of the wound together around the embedded object to control severe bleeding.
- If possible, raise and support the injured part of the body.

2 Cover wound

- Drape a piece of gauze gently over the wound and the protruding object to reduce the risk of infection.

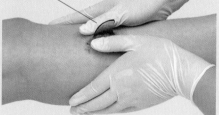

Press either side of wound

Gently lay gauze pad over embedded object

Raise injured part if possible

3 Pad around object

- Very carefully, place padding either side of the protruding object to protect the wound and control the bleeding.
- Build up enough padding so that you can bandage over the embedded object without pressing down on it.
- Make sure that you do not pull down on the embedded object as you position the padding.

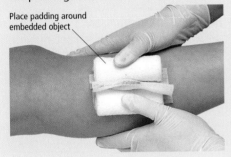

Place padding around embedded object

If the object does not protrude

- Place the padding either side of the object and wrap the bandage directly over the padding but without pressing down on the object.

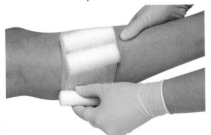

4 Bandage above and below object

- Place one end of a bandage over the part of the padding nearest to you.
- Make two straight turns with the bandage around the casualty's limb.
- Pass the bandage under the limb and wrap it around the other side of the padding.

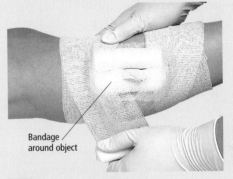

Bandage around object

5 Secure dressing

- Continue the diagonal turns around the injury on either side of the padding until the dressing is firm.
- Secure the bandage.
- Keep the injured part raised, where possible, and keep it as still as you can.
- Take or send the casualty to hospital.

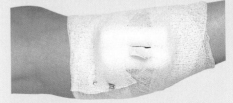

IMPORTANT
▶ Find out about the casualty's tetanus immunisations. Seek medical advice if the casualty has never had a tetanus injection, does not know when he was last injected or how many injections he has had, or it is more than 10 years since his last tetanus injection (p.62).

Splinters

Any tiny pieces or slivers of wood, glass, or metal that become embedded in the skin are rarely clean and may cause infection. If a splinter is sticking out of the skin, remove it with tweezers, as shown below. If the end of the splinter is not visible, seek medical help because it is easy to push a splinter even further into the skin.

Your aims	You will need
▶ Remove splinter from skin	▶ Disposable gloves
	▶ Cold water
▶ Prevent wound from becoming infected	▶ Tweezers
	▶ Match or lighter

SIGNS AND SYMPTOMS
▶ Pain where splinter went into skin
▶ Cause of injury may be close by
▶ Splinter visible in skin

1 Clean wound

● Put on disposable gloves, if available.
● Rinse the area around the splinter with cold water.
● Make sure that you do not touch the wound with your fingers.

Rinse away loose foreign particles with water

2 Sterilise tweezers

● Sterilise the tweezers by passing them through the flame of a match or lighter.
● Allow the tweezers to cool.
● Do not wipe the soot off or touch the end of the tweezers.

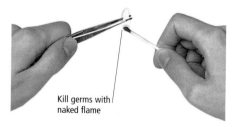

Kill germs with naked flame

3 Pull out splinter

● Grasp the splinter with the tweezers as close to the skin as possible.
● Carefully draw out the splinter, making sure that you pull it out at the same angle that it went into the skin.

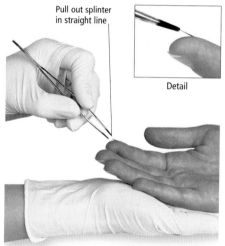

Pull out splinter in straight line

Detail

IMPORTANT
▶ Never dig into the skin to get at a splinter.
▶ If the splinter breaks, do not continue trying to remove it.
▶ Find out about the casualty's tetanus immunisations (p.62).

Fish-hook injury

When a fish-hook is embedded in the skin, do not try to remove it unless there is no medical help available. Simply bandage around the hook before making sure that the casualty receives medical help. Embedded fish-hooks carry a risk of infection.

Your aims	You will need
▶ Get medical help	▶ Disposable gloves
▶ Prevent further injury by padding around embedded fish-hook	▶ Scissors
	▶ Gauze pads
	▶ Bandage
If medical help is not available:	▶ Adhesive tape
▶ Remove hook	If medical help is not available:
	▶ Wirecutters
	▶ Sterile wound dressing

1 Help casualty sit down

● Help the casualty to sit in a comfortable position and reassure him.

2 Cut fishing line

● Put on disposable gloves, if available.
● Cut the fishing line as close as possible to the hook.

3 Build up pads of gauze

● Carefully put pads of gauze around the embedded fish-hook.
● Build up pads of gauze until you can bandage over the hook without pushing it further into the skin (pp.70–1).

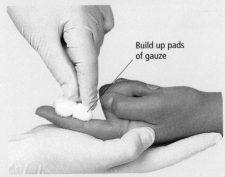
Build up pads of gauze

4 Bandage over gauze padding

● Bandage over the hook and padding, taking care not to press down on the hook.
● Secure the bandage with adhesive tape.
● Take or send the casualty to hospital

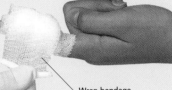
Wrap bandage over padding

If medical help is not available

Try to remove a fish-hook only if medical help is not available.
● If the barb of the hook is not visible, push it further into the skin until it pokes through.
● Cut off the barb with wirecutters.
● Never try to remove a fish-hook if you cannot cut off the barb as you will damage the underlying tissues.
● Withdraw the hook by its eye (the end that attaches to the fishing line).
● Clean the wound, and apply a sterile wound dressing and bandage.
● Find out about the casualty's tetanus immunisations (p.62).

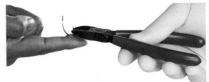

Test yourself

Now that you have read and studied the chapter on first-aid treatments for wounds and bleeding, see if you can answer the questions below. Check your answers against the correct ones on page 144.

1 Which three steps in the following list should you take to control bleeding?
  a Raise the wound above the level of the heart .... ☐
  b Give chest thrusts .... ☐
  c Apply pressure to the wound .... ☐
  d Cool the casualty with a wet sponge .... ☐
  e Apply a dressing and bandage to the wound .... ☐

2 What should you do if blood seeps through a dressing?
....
....

3 What are the three types of blood vessels that carry blood around the body?
1 ....
2 ....
3 ....

4 Which medical condition will develop if a large amount of blood is lost?
....
....

5 What should you do to prevent a graze becoming infected?
....
....
....
....
....
....

6 The first aider in the picture is monitoring someone with shock. What three things should she be checking?
1 ....
2 ....
3 ....

7 Why should you put a cold compress on a bruise?
....
....

8 What two actions should you tell a casualty with a nosebleed to do to stop the bleeding?
1 ....
2 ....

9 If you are unable to replant a knocked-out tooth in its socket, what should you do?
  a Place the tooth in the cheek until the casualty sees a dentist .... ☐
  b Keep the tooth in milk or water until the casualty sees a dentist .... ☐
  c Throw the tooth away .... ☐

10 If a yellowish, blood-stained fluid comes from the casualty's nose or ear, what might it indicate?
....

11 How do you control bleeding if there is an embedded object in a wound?
....
....
....
....

4 Environmental injuries

This chapter focuses on treating injuries and illnesses caused by environmental factors, such as extremes of heat and cold. Fire, electricity, hot liquids, and chemicals can all burn the skin, which protects the body and helps to maintain a normal body temperature. Extremes of temperature can also affect the skin and other body functions, especially in young children and elderly people.

This section of the book explains how to treat different types of burn and sets out the priorities for dealing with localised injuries, such as sunburn and frostbite, and generalised conditions, such as dehydration and heatstroke.

Use the questionnaire on page 88 to test your understanding of first aid for environmental injuries.

Contents

Dealing with severe burns	76
Types of burn	78
Minor burns and scalds	79
Face and head burns	80
Chemical burns	81
Electrical burns	82
Sunburn	83
Dehydration	84
Heat exhaustion	84
Heatstroke	85
Hypothermia	86
Frostbite	87
Test yourself	88

Dealing with severe burns

A burn or scald damages the skin and can lead to infection. Severe burns also cause loss of fluids, which will lead to shock (p.61). Scalds are burns caused by extremes of moist heat, such as boiling water or steam. When dealing with a burn, you need to act quickly to reduce the effect of the heat on the skin and prevent germs getting into the burnt area and causing infection. A severe burn requires urgent hospital treatment to minimise any subsequent damage (see When a casualty needs medical help p.78).

WARNING
▶ Any burning injury that is accompanied by smoke may lead to smoke inhalation and irritation of the airways and lungs, which may cause breathing difficulties.
▶ If the casualty is having breathing difficulties, be ready to begin resuscitation if necessary (pp.36–52).

Watch for shock
Look out for any signs of shock, such as pallor and sweating; the degree of shock will depend on the depth and extent of the burn

Get a history
Ask the casualty what caused the burn or scald

Cool burn
Flood burn with water

Blistered skin
If there are blisters, do not attempt to burst them because they provide a barrier to infection

Severe pain
The casualty will complain of pain if the surface of the skin is affected but deep burns are not usually painful because the nerve endings are destroyed

Swelling around injury
This will develop very quickly around any burn

Redness around injury
The skin will become red very quickly after an injury from a burn

Check for danger
Approach the casualty only if it is safe to do so. Check that whatever caused the incident represents no further danger to either of you

Give reassurance
Explain to the casualty what you are doing to help reassure her and keep her calm

What you should do

Your aims
▶ Cool burn
▶ Prevent infection
▶ Treat any shock
▶ Get medical help

IMPORTANT
▶ Do not apply creams, sprays, ointments, or adhesive tape.
▶ Do not touch the burnt area.
▶ Do not overcool as this may lead to hypothermia.
▶ Do not remove any clothing sticking to the burn.

1 Cool burn

● Flood the burn with copious amounts of cold water until the burning sensation eases.

2 Cover burn

● Put on disposable gloves, if available.
● Remove any burnt clothing unless it is sticking to the burn.
● Remove restrictions such as rings, bracelets, or belts before swelling starts.
● Cover the burnt area with a sterile wound dressing, clean cloth, plastic bag, or kitchen film to prevent infection.

3 Treat shock

● Watch for signs of shock developing and treat accordingly (p.61).
● Help the casualty to lie down.
● Constantly reassure the casualty.

4 Get medical help

● Seek urgent medical advice for all severe burns.
● Phone for an ambulance if necessary, or advise the casualty to see a doctor.
● Monitor the casualty's vital signs – level of response, pulse, and breathing (pp.20–1) – regularly until help arrives.

Make sure dressing is large enough to cover entire wound

Types of burn

The severity of a burn depends on the type of burn and on the size of the area of skin that is affected. There are three types of burn: superficial, partial-thickness, and full-thickness (below). A casualty with a full-thickness burn may not feel any pain because the nerve is damaged, which may make you and the casualty think that the burn is not as serious as it really is. Burns can cause fluid loss and lead to shock (p.61); the more extensive the burn, the greater the risk of shock. See the box below for detailed guidelines of when to get medical help for a burn. However, if you are in any doubt about the seriousness of a burn, always get medical advice.

How burns affect the skin

The skin is made up of two layers: the outermost visible layer called the epidermis and the inner dermis underneath. Skin has many functions, one of which is to protect the body from invasion by germs. A burn or scald can break this protective barrier, allowing germs to enter the body and lead to infection.

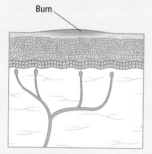

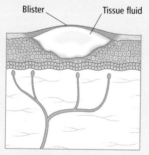

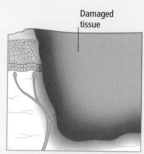

Superficial burn
This type of burn affects only the epidermis, causing redness and swelling. It is not serious unless it covers a large area (below). With prompt first aid, a superficial burn should heal in a few days.

Partial-thickness burn
This deeper burn destroys the epidermis. The skin turns red and is covered with blisters. This type of burn is painful but usually heals well. If, however, it covers a large area, it can be serious, even fatal.

Full-thickness burn
This type of burn destroys the epidermis and damages the dermis. It affects nerves, tissues, muscles, and blood vessels. The skin appears pale or charred. Full-thickness burns require urgent medical attention.

When a casualty needs medical help

Any infant or child with a burn should have urgent hospital treatment, regardless of the size of the burn. For adults, always seek medical help for any of the following:

- Full-thickness burns.
- Burns on the face, hands, feet, or genital area.
- Burns that reach right around an arm or a leg.
- Partial-thickness burns that cover an area about the size of the palm of the casualty's hand.
- Superficial burns that cover an area equivalent to the size of five of the casualty's palms.
- Burns of mixed depth.

Minor burns and scalds

The majority of small burns and scalds are the result of incidents in the kitchen. A burn may be caused by touching a hot oven or iron, while a scald may be the result of spilling boiling water on the skin or coming into contact with steam from a kettle.

Your aims	You will need
▶ Cool burn	▶ Cold water
▶ Relieve pain and swelling	▶ Disposable gloves
▶ Prevent burn from becoming infected	▶ Sterile wound dressing

SIGNS AND SYMPTOMS
▶ Reddening of skin
▶ Pain in area of burn
▶ Blister, smaller than casualty's palm

IMPORTANT
▶ If you are at all concerned about the severity of the burn, make sure the casualty gets medical help.

1 Cool burn

● Flood the area of the burn with copious quantities of cold water for at least 10 minutes or until the burning feeling stops.
● If water is not available, use any cold liquid, such as canned drinks.

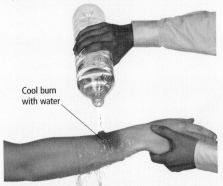

Cool burn with water

3 Cover burn

● Cover the burn with a sterile wound dressing or a clean, non-fluffy pad (p.24) to minimise the risk of infection. Alternatively cover the burn with a clean plastic bag, clean tea towel, clean sheet, or kitchen film. Discard the first piece of film to make sure the film you use to cover the burn is as clean as possible.
● Tie the bandage loosely over the dressing to hold it in place.

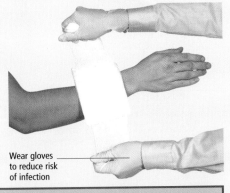

2 Raise limb

● Put on disposable gloves, if available.
● Raise the limb to reduce swelling.
● Remove any constricting jewellery or clothing before the area starts to swell.

Wear gloves to reduce risk of infection

WARNING
▶ Do not put any lotions, creams, ointments, or sprays on the burn as they might introduce infection.
▶ Do not put on any dressing that will stick to the burnt area because it will be difficult to remove without causing further damage.

▶ Do not burst any blisters or touch the burnt area. A small blister does not usually need any treatment, but if it bursts, apply a non-adhesive sterile wound dressing that extends beyond the edges of the blister. Leave the dressing in place until the blister heals.

Face and head burns

Burns to the face, and in the mouth or throat, are particularly serious because they can cause the casualty's airway to become swollen very quickly, making breathing difficult. If the burns are in the mouth or throat, you can usually see external signs of burning, such as soot around the mouth. For all these burns, emergency medical help is vital.

Your aims	You will need
▶ Get casualty to hospital urgently	▶ Cold water
▶ Keep airway open	▶ Towel
▶ Treat for shock if necessary	▶ Disposable gloves
	▶ Sterile wound dressing

SIGNS AND SYMPTOMS

▶ Very painful mouth, throat, and head
▶ Difficulty breathing
▶ Damaged skin and/or soot around mouth
▶ Shock may develop

WARNING

▶ If the casualty is unconscious, open the airway and check breathing. Put him in the recovery position if he is breathing. Be ready to begin resuscitation if necessary (pp.36–52).

1 Call an ambulance

- Phone for an ambulance immediately.
- Tell the control officer that you suspect burns to the airway and that the casualty is having difficulty breathing.

2 Improve air supply

- Do anything you can to improve the casualty's air supply, such as loosening tight clothing around the neck.
- Treat for shock, if necessary (p.61).

Burns to the head

- Keep the burnt area cool; if possible, use a bottle or watering can or something similar to pour water gently over the head. Put a towel around the shoulders to catch the water.
- If the burn is near the throat, nose, or mouth, be ready to begin resuscitation (pp.36–52).
- Put on disposable gloves, if available, and place a dressing on the burn but do not bandage it in place; if necessary, hold the dressing on until help arrives.

Undo buttons at neck to help breathing

Chemical burns

Many chemicals used in the home, in the workshop, or in industry can cause serious damage to the skin. Always act quickly to wash the chemical off and protect yourself as you treat the casualty. Make sure any contaminated water can drain away freely.

Your aims	You will need	SIGNS AND SYMPTOMS
▶ Wash chemical away	▶ Disposable gloves	▶ Chemicals near casualty
▶ Get casualty to hospital	▶ Cold water	▶ Stinging pain
	▶ Sterile wound dressing	▶ Discoloration, swelling, and blistering of skin
		▶ Shock may develop

1 Wash chemical off skin

● Put on disposable gloves, if available.
● Hold the injured part under cold running water for at least 20 minutes to wash away the chemical.
● Take any contaminated clothing off the casualty while you are flooding the affected area with water.

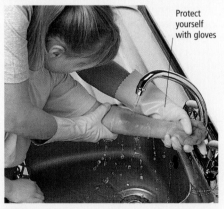

Protect yourself with gloves

2 Cover wound

● After washing the area, cover the burn with a sterile wound dressing.
● If necessary, treat the casualty for shock (p.61).

✚ **TAKE OR SEND CASUALTY TO HOSPITAL**

Burns to the eye

If the casualty has been splashed in the eye with a chemical, his eye will water and the surrounding area will become swollen. He may also not be able to open his eye. Act quickly to wash the chemical out of the casualty's eye.

● Put on disposable gloves, if available.
● Positioning the head so that contaminated water does not run down the face, hold the affected eye under gently running cold water for at least 10 minutes.
● If the casualty is still in pain, continue pouring water over the eye.
● Take or send the casualty to hospital.
● Once the pain has eased, ask the casualty to hold a sterile wound dressing lightly over the eye.

Position head so affected eye is under tap

Make sure contaminated water drains away from face

Electrical burns

These burns can occur when an electrical current passes through the body and may be visible at the point where electricity enters or leaves the body. Electrical burns at home are caused by low-voltage current, so it is safe to switch the current off; do not approach a person who has suffered high-voltage burns (p.11).

Your aims	You will need
▶ Treat visible burns and any shock	▶ Cold water
▶ Get casualty to hospital urgently	▶ Sterile wound dressing or clean, non-fluffy material
	▶ Scissors

SIGNS AND SYMPTOMS
- ▶ Casualty may be unconscious
- ▶ Swollen, charred skin at site of contact
- ▶ Shock may develop
- ▶ High-voltage burn may leave brownish residue on skin

1 Turn off electricity

● Where possible, turn off the electricity at the mains or meter point to break the contact between the casualty and the electrical supply. Alternatively, pull out the plug from the socket.

2 Cool burn

● Pour cold water over the burn for at least 10 minutes or until the burning feeling stops.
● Carefully cut away any clothing from around the burn.

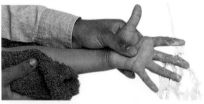

3 Cover burn

● Place a sterile wound dressing carefully over the burn.
● If you do not have a wound dressing, place some clean, non-fluffy material, such as a clean, folded triangular bandage or kitchen film, over the affected area or put a clean plastic bag over a burnt hand or foot, securing the bag with tape.

✚ CALL AN AMBULANCE

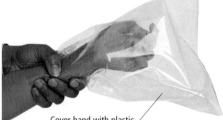

Cover hand with plastic bag if no wound dressing available

4 Reassure casualty

● Reassure the casualty and, if necessary, treat for shock (p.61).

IMPORTANT
▶ If the casualty has suffered a high-voltage burn (p.11), do not approach him until the current has been officially switched off. Keep yourself and bystanders at a safe distance of 18m (60ft) from the source of electricity.

WARNING
▶ Do not touch the casualty if you cannot break the contact as you may be electrocuted. Follow the advice given on p.11.
▶ An electrical burn may cause internal damage and lead to unconsciousness. If the casualty is unconscious, open the airway and check his breathing. Put him in the recovery position if he is breathing. Be ready to begin resuscitation if necessary (pp.36–52).

✚ CALL AN AMBULANCE

Sunburn

Over-exposure to the sun's rays will result in sunburn. At high altitudes, it is possible to get sunburnt even if the sky is overcast; reflected off snow, the effects of sunlight are intensified and particularly damaging. Using a sunlamp may also cause sunburn. If a casualty is severely sunburnt, he may also suffer from heatstroke (p.85).

Your aims	You will need
▶ Take casualty out of sun ▶ Relieve discomfort and pain	▶ Cold water and towel/sponge ▶ Drinking water ▶ Calamine lotion/after-sun cream

SIGNS AND SYMPTOMS
▶ Red and very hot skin
▶ Superficial burns
▶ Blistering
▶ Heatstroke

IMPORTANT
Prevention is better than cure:
▶ Wear sunscreen when in the sun.
▶ Do not stay in the sun for too long.
▶ Limit exposure to the sun by wearing a hat, and uncover only small areas of the body at a time.

1 Take casualty into shade

● Cover the casualty's skin with light clothing or a towel and move him out of the sun and into the shade.

2 Cool burn

● Remove the clothing.
● Cool the burnt area by gently dabbing on cold water with a towel or sponge.

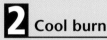
Cool burnt areas

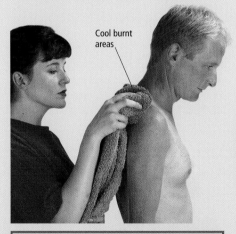

3 Give water

● Give the casualty frequent sips of water.

Make sure casualty sips water

4 Apply soothing lotion

● If the sunburn is mild, apply calamine or after-sun cream to the skin.

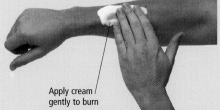
Apply cream gently to burn

WARNING
▶ If the skin is blistered or the sunburn covers a large area,

✚ **TAKE OR SEND CASUALTY TO HOSPITAL**

Dehydration

Water makes up 50–60 per cent of the body of a healthy adult. Normally, there is a balance between the amount of water the body takes in and the amount the body excretes. Dehydration occurs when the body has too little water. It is common in babies who are ill, elderly people, and those suffering from diarrhoea, vomiting, or a fever. Exercise, particularly if it is strenuous or takes place in hot weather, can result in dehydration.

Your aims	You will need
▶ Replace water ▶ Treat cause ▶ Get medical help if necessary	▶ Drinking water, preferably non-fizzy ▶ Notepad and pen

SIGNS AND SYMPTOMS
▶ Feeling thirsty
▶ Nausea
▶ Muscle cramps

1 Give sips of water

● Give the casualty frequent small sips of water to replace lost body fluids. Continue until he stops feeling thirsty. If possible, use only still water, not fizzy.

2 Find cause of dehydration

● Look for any other illness, such as fever or vomiting and diarrhoea, to try to discover why the casualty is dehydrated.
● Prevent any strenuous exercise until the casualty has recovered.

3 Monitor casualty

● Monitor and record the casualty's vital signs – level of response, pulse, and breathing (pp.20–1) – regularly.
● If the casualty does not recover or his condition worsens, get medical help.

Heat exhaustion

This condition is caused by an abnormal loss of salt and water from the body through excessive sweating. It usually develops gradually and is more likely to affect people who are not accustomed to hot and humid conditions and those who are already ill.

Your aims	You will need
▶ Cool casualty down ▶ Replace lost fluid ▶ Get casualty to hospital urgently	▶ Drinking water or non-fizzy drink

SIGNS AND SYMPTOMS
▶ Cramp-like pains and/or headache
▶ Pale, moist skin
▶ Fast, weak pulse
▶ Slightly raised temperature

1 Help casualty lie down

● Help the casualty to lie down in a cool place.
● Raise his legs to improve blood flow.

2 Give water

● Give the casualty plenty of water to drink or a non-fizzy drink to replace lost fluids.

✚ **CALL AN AMBULANCE**

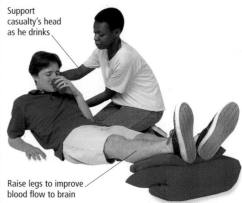

Support casualty's head as he drinks

Raise legs to improve blood flow to brain

Heatstroke

This potentially dangerous condition occurs when the body is unable to cool itself by sweating, due to illness or prolonged exposure to heat and humidity. The use of drugs such as ecstasy can raise the body temperature and may lead to heatstroke. Common in tropical areas, the condition can also occur during hot spells in milder climates. People who exercise in hot weather are particularly prone to heatstroke.

Your aims	You will need	SIGNS AND SYMPTOMS
▶ Lower casualty's body temperature as quickly as possible ▶ Get casualty to hospital urgently	▶ Cushions/pillows ▶ Two large sheets ▶ Water and spray ▶ Fan (preferably electric but keep away from water) ▶ Thermometer ▶ Notepad and pen	▶ Restlessness ▶ Headache ▶ Dizzy feeling ▶ Flushed and very hot skin ▶ Rapid loss of consciousness ▶ Fast, strong pulse ▶ Raised body temperature, which may reach 40°C (104°F) or higher

1 Get casualty to cool place

● Help the casualty to lie down in a cool place and remove his outer clothes.
● Place cushions or pillows behind his head to make him more comfortable.

2 Cool with water and fan

● If available, wrap the casualty in a cold, wet sheet and keep it wet, or sponge his body down with cold or tepid water.
✚ CALL AN AMBULANCE
● Fan the casualty until his temperature falls to 38°C (100.4°F) under the tongue, or 37.5°C (99.5°F) under the armpit (p.21).

3 Change sheet

● When the casualty's temperature has fallen to a safe level, replace the wet sheet with a dry one.

4 Monitor casualty

● Monitor and record his vital signs – level of response, pulse, and breathing (pp.20–1) – regularly until help arrives.

Make casualty comfortable with cushions or pillows

Spray sheet continually with water to keep it wet

Wrap casualty in wet sheet

Hypothermia

When the body temperature drops below 35°C (95°F), hypothermia sets in. It is often caused by wearing unsuitable clothes in cold weather or by being in cold water for too long. It can also result from being in a poorly heated or unheated room. Elderly people are especially at risk because they are less aware of changes in temperature. Infants, too, are susceptible to hypothermia because they are not capable of regulating their own body temperatures. For a casualty with hypothermia outdoors, treat as described below. For a casualty with hypothermia indoors, see opposite.

Your aims	You will need	SIGNS AND SYMPTOMS
▶ Prevent casualty's body temperature falling any further	▶ Warm, dry clothes	▶ Loss of consciousness
▶ Make casualty warmer	▶ Blankets, survival bag, or sleeping bag	▶ Very cold, pale skin
▶ Get medical help if necessary	▶ Insulating material, such as bracken	▶ Shivering
	▶ Warm drink	▶ Clumsiness, irritability
		▶ Slurred speech
		▶ Slow breathing, weak pulse, and lethargy

1 Rewarm casualty

● Advise the casualty to stop any physical activity immediately and rest.
● If possible, remove any wet clothing and replace with warm, dry clothes.
● Insulate the casualty with extra clothing and blankets.
● If possible, send someone to get help.

2 Shelter casualty

● If possible, make a shelter to protect the casualty from the weather.
● Wrap her in a survival bag, sleeping bag, or blanket.
● Lay her down on dry, insulating material, such as dry heather or bracken.

Protect casualty from wind and rain with a survival bag

3 Give casualty warm drink

● If possible, give the casualty a warm drink, such as warmed milk or cocoa. Do not give her alcohol.
● Reassure and comfort her.

Give casualty a warm drink

4 Check for frostbite

● If the casualty appears to have frostbite (opposite), treat her accordingly.

5 Get casualty to hospital

● Arrange to get the casualty to hospital – she must be carried on a stretcher. Do not let her walk or leave her alone.

WARNING
▶ If the casualty is unconscious, open the airway and check breathing. Put her in the recovery position if she is breathing. Be ready to begin resuscitation if necessary (pp.36–52).

For a casualty indoors

● If a casualty has been brought inside wearing wet clothes, replace these with warm, dry clothes as soon as possible.
● If the casualty is young and fit and can climb into a bath on her own, rewarm her in the bath, making sure the water temperature is not too hot – about 40°C (104°F).
● If the casualty is elderly or an infant, wrap her in blankets to rewarm her.
● Put the warmed casualty into bed and make sure she is well covered. Cover her head for additional warmth.
● Do not use a hot-water bottle or an electric blanket to warm a casualty.
● Give warm drinks, soup, or high-energy foods, such as chocolate, to help rewarm the casualty. Do not give any alcohol to drink because this will make the hypothermia worse.

✚ GET MEDICAL HELP

● Stay with the casualty until her skin becomes warm and returns to its normal colour.

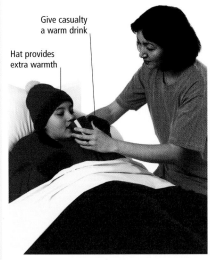

Give casualty a warm drink

Hat provides extra warmth

Frostbite

Intense cold causes frostbite, resulting in parts of the body, such as the fingers or toes, becoming frozen. It may be accompanied by hypothermia (opposite).

SIGNS AND SYMPTOMS
▶ Prickling pain, followed by gradual loss of feeling
▶ Skin feels hard and turns white, then blue, and finally black

Your aims	You will need
▶ Warm affected area slowly ▶ Get casualty to hospital	▶ Gauze bandage

1 Warm affected area

● Gently remove any tight or constrictive clothing, such as gloves or boots, as well as any rings, from around the affected part.
● Get the casualty to put his hands in his armpits or put his feet in your armpits.

2 Cover affected area

● Cover the frostbitten part with a gauze bandage to protect it.
● Keep the area covered until colour and feeling return to the skin.

✚ TAKE OR SEND CASUALTY TO HOSPITAL

IMPORTANT
▶ Warm the affected part slowly to prevent further tissue damage.
▶ Do not warm the frostbitten part with a hot-water bottle.
▶ Do not thaw a frostbitten foot if the casualty needs to walk any further.

Test yourself

Now that you have read and studied the chapter on first-aid treatments for environmental injuries, see if you can answer the questions below. Check your answers against the correct ones on page 144.

1 What are your aims when treating a burn?

....
....
....

2 Name the three types of burn.

1 ....
2 ....
3 ....

3 What is the greatest risk from extensive burns?

....
....

4 When treating a burn, what should you not do?

....
....
....
....

5 Suggest some household items that can be used to cover a burn if you do not have a sterile wound dressing or pad.

....
....
....

6 What external signs might indicate burns to the mouth or throat?

....
....
....

7 How long should you cool a burn caused by heat and what is the risk to the casualty of cooling it for too long?

....
....
....

8 How long should a chemical burn to the skin be held under cold running water?

....
....

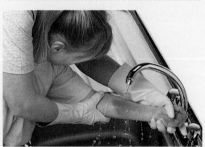

9 What should your first action be when treating an electrical burn?

....
....

10 An athlete is feeling unwell after running a half-marathon on a hot summer's day. What might be the problem?

....
....

11 Name at least five signs or symptoms that indicate that a casualty has hypothermia.

1 ....
2 ....
3 ....
4 ....
5 ....

12 What are your aims when treating a casualty with frostbite?

....
....
....

5 Disorders affecting consciousness

This chapter describes first aid for injuries or conditions that affect consciousness. It begins by outlining the first-aid priorities for dealing with someone who has collapsed, explaining why it is important to carefully monitor a casualty who is not fully conscious.

Easy-to-follow anatomical information helps you understand the effects that impaired consciousness can have on the body. This is followed by first-aid guidelines for the injuries or conditions that can lead to loss of consciousness: head injury, stroke (in which there is bleeding or a blood clot in the brain), fainting (which happens when insufficient oxygen-rich blood reaches the brain), and seizures (in which there is an electrical imbalance in the brain).

Use the questionnaire on page 100 to test your understanding of first aid for disorders affecting consciousness.

Contents

Dealing with a collapsed person   90

The nervous system   92

Head injury   93

Concussion   94

Compression   95

Stroke   96

Fainting   97

Epilepsy   98

Seizures in children   99

Test yourself   100

Dealing with a collapsed person

Some injuries and illnesses can result in a casualty becoming dazed, confused, or even unconscious. The casualty may be wide awake and alert, completely unresponsive to outside stimulation, or somewhere between these two extremes. If you are dealing with a casualty who is not fully conscious, monitor any change in her level of response (p.20), especially any deterioration, because she could become unconscious at any time.

IMPORTANT

▶ If you suspect the casualty has a neck or spinal injury, try to leave her in the position in which you found her. If you need to place her in the recovery position (p.38 adults; p.47 children), keep her head and neck in alignment with the body.

Get a history
If the casualty is alert enough, ask what happened. If the casualty is not alert, ask any bystanders what happened and listen carefully to what they say

Speak to the casualty
Does she respond to simple questions or is she confused and unable to speak clearly?

Look for external clues
Check for clues such as a special bracelet or necklace, worn by people with conditions that may affect the level of consciousness, for example epilepsy or diabetes mellitus

Check breathing
Note whether the casualty's breathing is noisy, difficult, or apparently normal

Look at her eyes
Assess how alert the casualty is by checking if her eyes are open and moving

Check for danger
Look out for any hazards before helping the casualty. Approach her only when you are sure that you are not in any danger

WARNING
▶ If the casualty becomes unconscious, be ready to begin resuscitation if necessary (pp.36–52).

Find cause of injury
Visually examine the casualty from head to toe. Look for an obvious cause of injury or a pre-existing condition. For example, check whether she has fallen against something that may have caused a head injury

What you should do

Your aims
▶ Assess casualty's level of consciousness and monitor any change
▶ Look for possible causes
▶ Arrange removal to hospital if necessary

IMPORTANT
▶ Do not leave casualty unless you have to go for help.
▶ Do not move casualty unnecessarily.
▶ Do not allow casualty to eat, drink, or smoke.
▶ Do not shake an infant or child.

1 Check response
● Assess the casualty's level of response by following the AVPU code (p.20).
● If the casualty is unconscious, call for help, open the airway, check breathing, and be ready to begin resuscitation if necessary (pp.36–52).
● If the casualty is conscious, ask her what happened or if she has any known injury or illness.

2 Check her breathing
● Note the rate, depth, and quality of the casualty's breathing (p.21).
● Listen especially for breathing difficulties.

3 Help casualty sit or lie down
● Help the casualty to sit or lie down in a comfortable position. If she is very dazed, help her to lie down rather than sit her in a chair because she may fall off the chair.

4 Do head-to-toe survey
● Examine the casualty from head to toe for any injuries or illnesses (pp.18–19) and treat them accordingly.
● Look for warning signs, such as a special bracelet or necklace indicating a pre-existing condition.
● Call an ambulance if necessary.

5 Monitor casualty
● Monitor and record the casualty's vital signs – level of response, pulse, and breathing (pp.20–1) – regularly until help arrives.

Check pulse at wrist

The nervous system

This is the system that controls body functions, such as consciousness, breathing, and movement, as well as detecting and responding to information coming from outside and inside the body. The nervous system consists of the brain and spinal cord (central nervous system) and a network of nerves branching from this system (peripheral nervous system). Any injury or illness that affects the nervous system is potentially serious because it may affect a casualty's level of consciousness.

How the nervous system works

The brain contains millions of interconnected nerve cells, which control thought, sensation, movement, and functions such as breathing. The main function of the spinal cord is to convey high-speed electrical signals between the brain and the "wire-like" peripheral nerves.

    The peripheral system has three divisions: sensory nerves that send information to the brain and spinal cord from sensory cells, for example in the eyes, ears, and skin; motor nerves that carry signals from the brain that allow us to move our muscles voluntarily; and autonomic nerves, which control involuntary, or "automatic", body functions, such as breathing, heartbeat, and digestion.

Brain

Peripheral nerve from brain

Spinal cord

Peripheral nerve from spinal cord

Cerebrospinal fluid circulates around brain and spinal cord and acts as a shock absorber

Cerebrum

Skull

Cerebellum

Brainstem

Spinal cord

Functions of the brain
The brain interprets information that it receives from the body. The cerebrum controls voluntary responses, such as walking and thought. The cerebellum controls balance and posture. Involuntary responses, such as breathing and heartbeat, are controlled by the brainstem. The brain and spinal cord are bathed in a nourishing fluid called cerebrospinal fluid and surrounded by protective membranes called meninges.

Structure of the nervous system
The nervous system consists of the brain, spinal cord, and a dense network of nerves that carries information in the form of electrical signals between the brain and the rest of the body.

Head injury

Any blow to the head can cause a fracture of the skull and/or concussion or bleeding inside the skull leading to compression of the brain. If the casualty shows any of the signs and symptoms that are listed below or on pages 94 and 95, the injury may be life-threatening. Get emergency medical help. Treat a conscious casualty as described below. For an unconscious casualty, see the box below.

Your aims	You will need
▶ Assess casualty carefully	▶ Notepad and pen
▶ Get medical help	

SIGNS AND SYMPTOMS
▶ Period of unconsciousness
▶ Yellowish, blood-stained fluid from ear or nose
▶ Bruising around eyelid or white part of eye
▶ Bleeding scalp
▶ Exposed skull
▶ Enlarged or different-sized pupils
▶ Unusually slow pulse rate

1 Check responses

● Check the casualty's level of response using the AVPU code (p.20).
● If the casualty is conscious and responsive, help her to sit or lie in a comfortable position. Continue to monitor her level of response.

Ask a simple question

IMPORTANT
▶ Always suspect a spinal injury (p.110) with anyone who has had a head injury.

2 Get medical help

● Advise the casualty to seek medical help if she later develops a headache, blurred vision, nausea, or excessive sleepiness.
● If the casualty does not recover fully or if, after an initial recovery, her level of response deteriorates, call an ambulance.
● If there is a yellowish, blood-stained fluid coming from the nose or ear, suspect a skull facture and call an ambulance.

For an unconscious casualty

● If possible, leave the casualty in the position in which you found her.
● Open her airway using the jaw-thrust method (see For an unconscious casualty p.111), in case she has a spinal injury, and check her breathing. Be ready to begin resuscitation if necessary (pp.36–52).
● If there are any bystanders present, ask one to call an ambulance.

● If the casualty is breathing and you need to leave her to call an ambulance, put her in the recovery position (p.38 adults; p.47 children; p.51 infants).
● Monitor and record her vital signs – level of response, pulse, and breathing (pp.20–1) – regularly until help arrives.
● If she makes a rapid recovery, check her responses every 10 minutes and watch for signs of deterioration.

Concussion

This is usually caused by a blow to the head, which "shakes" the brain inside the skull, but it can also result from indirect force, such as landing heavily on your feet. The casualty will be dazed and confused but probably for only a few minutes. Concussion is always followed by a complete recovery. If the casualty later complains of symptoms such as a headache or blurred vision, advise her to seek medical help.

Your aims	You will need
▶ Make sure casualty recovers fully ▶ Get casualty looked after by responsible person ▶ Get medical help	▶ Notepad and pen

SIGNS AND SYMPTOMS
▶ Blow to head
▶ Short period of being dazed and confused
▶ Dizziness
▶ Nausea
▶ Brief loss of memory
▶ Headache

1 Help casualty sit or lie down

● Help the casualty to sit or lie down in a comfortable position.

IMPORTANT
▶ Always suspect a spinal injury (p.110) with anyone who has had a head injury.

2 Check responses

● Check the casualty's level of response using the AVPU code (p.20).
● Monitor and record her vital signs – level of response, pulse, and breathing (pp.20–1) – regularly. Pay particular attention to her level of response.
● Treat any associated injuries.

3 Stay with casualty

● When the casualty has recovered, make sure someone responsible stays with her for the next few hours.
● If the injury has occurred during a sporting activity, do not allow her to continue playing the sport without first getting medical advice.

4 Get medical help

● Advise the casualty to seek medical help if she later suffers from a persistent headache, nausea and vomiting, blurred vision, or excessive sleepiness.

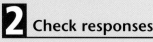

Check casualty's pulse

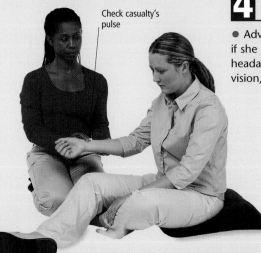

WARNING
▶ If the casualty does not recover completely after a short time, if her level of response deteriorates after an initial recovery, or if there is an accompanying neck or other serious injury,

✚ CALL AN AMBULANCE

Compression

A heavy blow to the head can cause bleeding inside the skull or swelling of the injured part of the brain. This disturbs the brain's normal activity, resulting in a very serious, life-threatening condition known as cerebral compression. The casualty will probably need urgent medical or surgical treatment. Treat a conscious casualty as described below. For an unconscious casualty, see the box at the bottom of the page.

Your aims	You will need
▶ Get casualty to hospital urgently ▶ Reassure casualty ▶ Monitor casualty	▶ Notepad and pen

1 Call an ambulance

● Phone for an ambulance immediately.

2 Help casualty sit or lie down

● Help the conscious casualty to sit or lie down in a comfortable position and reassure her.

3 Monitor casualty

● Monitor and record the casualty's vital signs – level of response, pulse, and breathing (pp.20–1) – regularly until help arrives.

SIGNS AND SYMPTOMS
▶ Deteriorating level of response
▶ History of head injury
▶ Severe headache
▶ Unequal pupil size
▶ Weakness and/or paralysis down one side of body or face
▶ Change in behaviour
▶ Noisy breathing
▶ Slow, strong pulse
▶ High temperature and flushed face

WARNING
▶ Compression may develop immediately after a head injury, a few hours later, or even days later.
▶ Compression can also be caused by a stroke (p.96), brain tumour, or infection.

IMPORTANT
▶ Always suspect a spinal injury (p.110) with anyone who has had a head injury.
▶ Do not let the casualty eat, drink, or smoke – she may need a general anaesthetic later in hospital.

For an unconscious casualty

● If possible, leave the casualty in the position in which you found her.
● Open her airway using the jaw-thrust method (see For an unconscious casualty p.111), and check her breathing. Be ready to begin resuscitation if necessary (pp.36–52).
● If there are any bystanders present, ask one to call an ambulance.
● If the casualty is breathing and you need to leave her to call an ambulance, put her in the recovery position (p.38 adults; p.47 children; p.51 infants).

● Monitor and record her vital signs – level of response, pulse, and breathing (pp.20–1) – regularly until help arrives.

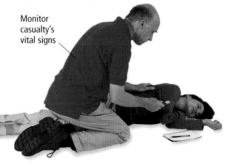

Monitor casualty's vital signs

Stroke

A stroke occurs when the flow of blood in the brain is disrupted by a clot or bleeding from a damaged blood vessel. Strokes can be minor, in which case a full recovery is possible, or they can be major and possibly fatal. The severity of the stroke depends on the extent of the damage and where in the brain it has occurred. If you suspect a person has suffered a stroke, call an ambulance immediately. Treat a conscious casualty as described below. For an unconscious casualty, see the box at the bottom of the page.

Your aims	You will need
▶ Keep casualty comfortable	▶ Damp flannel
▶ Get casualty to hospital urgently	▶ Notepad and pen

SIGNS AND SYMPTOMS
▶ Severe, sudden headache
▶ Dizziness and confusion
▶ Gradual or sudden loss of consciousness
▶ Paralysis down one side of body, with weak limbs and drooping of one side of face

1 Support head and shoulders

● Help the casualty to lie down.
● Make sure her head and shoulders are slightly raised.

IMPORTANT
▶ Do not allow the casualty to have anything to eat or drink because she may choke.

2 Tilt casualty's head

● Tilt the casualty's head towards the weaker side to allow fluid to drain out.
● Wipe her face with a damp flannel if she dribbles.

✚ CALL AN AMBULANCE

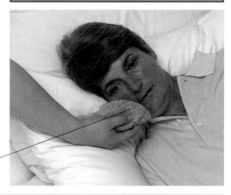

Wipe away saliva with damp flannel

For an unconscious casualty

● Open the casualty's airway and check breathing. Put her in the recovery position if she is breathing, making sure her airway stays open. Be ready to begin resuscitation if necessary (pp.36–52).

✚ CALL AN AMBULANCE
● Monitor and record her vital signs – level of response, pulse, and breathing (pp.20–1) – regularly until help arrives.

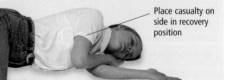

Place casualty on side in recovery position

Fainting

A person faints when the amount of blood flowing to the brain is temporarily reduced, leading to a brief loss of consciousness. This can be caused by excessive pain but it can be the result of extreme emotion or standing still for a long time in a hot atmosphere – moving the feet and/or changing position can prevent this. If you give the correct first aid, the casualty will usually recover quickly and completely.

Your aims
▶ Make sure blood reaches brain
▶ Make casualty comfortable
▶ Reassure casualty after recovery

SIGNS AND SYMPTOMS
▶ Feeling weak, faint, giddy, and possibly nauseous
▶ Very pale skin
▶ Slow pulse
▶ Loss of consciousness

WARNING
▶ If the casualty does not recover quickly, put her in the recovery position (p.38 adults; p.47 children; p.51 infants) and
✚ CALL AN AMBULANCE

1 Raise legs above heart

● Help the casualty to lie down.
● If she has already fainted, open her airway and check her breathing (p.37).
● Raise her legs above heart (chest) level.

Raise legs above heart level

Loosen tight clothing

2 Get fresh air to casualty

● Loosen tight clothing around the neck, chest, and waist.
● Open any windows and ask bystanders not to crowd the casualty.

3 Reassure casualty

● Once the casualty starts to recover, reassure her constantly and help her to sit up slowly.
● Treat any associated injuries.

Epilepsy

The most likely cause of a person suffering from a seizure is epilepsy, which is the result of electrical activity in the brain being disturbed. Epileptic seizures may be sudden and dramatic (below) or quite minor, with the casualty looking as if she is daydreaming. Many epileptics carry a warning card or wear a Medic-Alert bracelet.

Your aims	You will need
▶ Protect casualty from injury ▶ Reassure casualty when she recovers	▶ Soft padding, such as towel/pillow

SIGNS AND SYMPTOMS
▶ Sudden loss of consciousness
▶ Rigid body
▶ Convulsive jerking movements
▶ Relaxation of muscles at end of attack

1 Clear space around casualty

● If possible, try to ease the casualty's fall.
● Clear a space around her so that she does not hurt herself, and protect her from any danger.
● Keep calm and let the seizure run its course; there is nothing you can do to stop it.

2 Protect head

● If possible, place padding, such as towels or pillows, under or around her head to prevent injury (do this very carefully as it is easy to frighten someone who is having a seizure).
● Carefully loosen any tight clothing.

3 Place in recovery position

● When the jerking stops, open the airway and check the breathing.
● Put her in the recovery position (p.38 adults; p.47 children; p.51 infants).

4 Reassure casualty

● After the attack, remain with the casualty until she has fully recovered. Monitor and record her vital signs (pp.20–1) regularly.

WARNING
▶ If the seizure lasts more than 5 minutes, if unconsciousness lasts more than 10 minutes, if the casualty has repeated seizures and/or she does not regain consciousness, or if this is her first seizure,

✚ CALL AN AMBULANCE

IMPORTANT
▶ Do not try to hold the casualty down or stop the seizure.
▶ Do not put anything in the mouth.
▶ Do not give the casualty anything to eat or drink during a seizure.

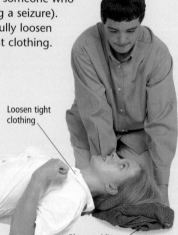

Loosen tight clothing

Place padding under head

Seizures in children

Young children tend to suffer from seizures when they are between the ages of one and four. They are generally caused by a high temperature (fever), serious tummy upset, fright, or temper. Although seizures can look very alarming, they are not usually dangerous, and problems rarely occur afterwards.

Your aims	You will need
▶ Protect child from injury	▶ Soft padding, such as towel/pillow
▶ Prevent temperature from rising further	▶ Notepad and pen
▶ Get child to hospital urgently	

SIGNS AND SYMPTOMS
▶ Flushed and sweating face
▶ Very hot forehead
▶ Stiffening and arching of back
▶ Eyes rolled upwards
▶ Child may hold breath, resulting in bluish tinge to face
▶ Brief loss of consciousness

1 Protect child

● Place padding such as towels or pillows around the child to prevent her from injuring herself by a sudden movement.

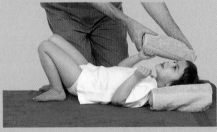

2 Cool child

● Remove the child's clothing and any bedclothes to prevent her temperature from rising further.
● Make sure there is a good supply of cool fresh air around her.

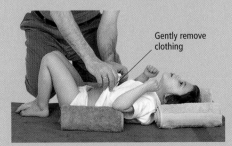

Gently remove clothing

3 Cover with sheet

● When the seizure stops, help the child to lie on her side if possible. Cover her with a sheet.
● Reassure her.

✚ CALL AN AMBULANCE

● Monitor and record the child's vital signs – level of response, pulse, and breathing (pp.20–1) – regularly until help arrives.

Put sheet over child

IMPORTANT
▶ Take care not to overcool the child.
▶ If the child loses consciousness, put her in the recovery position (p.47).

✚ CALL AN AMBULANCE

Test yourself

Now that you have read and studied the chapter on first-aid treatments for disorders affecting consciousness, see if you can answer the questions below. Check your answers against the correct ones on page 144.

1 Why are injuries that affect the brain a cause for concern?
....
....

2 What five conditions might any head injury be accompanied by?
1..
2..
3..
4..
5..

3 How would you recognise compression?
....
....

4 How would you recognise concussion?
....
....

5 What should you do if a casualty becomes unconscious?
....
....
....

6 Which of the following can cause a stroke?
  a A blood clot in an artery
  in the heart ....☐
  b A blood clot in an artery
  in the brain ....☐
  c Bleeding from a damaged
  blood vessel in the brain ....☐
  d A blood clot in the lungs..................☐

7 What is fainting?
....
....

8 Which of the following should you do when a casualty is having an epileptic seizure?
  a Make sure the casualty's
  mouth is kept open ....☐
  b Try to give the casualty
  a sip of cool water............................☐
  c Clear a space around the casualty
  so that he does not hurt himself ....☐
  d Send the casualty back to work
  as soon as the seizure is over. ....☐
  e Try to hold the casualty tightly ....☐

9 What are the three most important actions to take when a child is having a seizure?
1..
2..
3..

10 If you are waiting for medical help to arrive, what three things should you monitor regularly until it arrives?
1..
2..
3..

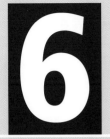

6 Bone, joint, and muscle injuries

This chapter describes first aid for injuries that affect the bones, joints, and the muscles that move them. The section begins by outlining your priorities for dealing with a suspected broken bone, because it can be very difficult for a first aider to differentiate between the different types of injury and this is the safest course of action.

There are easy-to-follow descriptions of the potential injuries: broken bones, sprained joints, dislocated joints, and strained muscles. This is followed by first-aid procedures for injuries to different parts of the body, from a broken jaw and cheekbone to rib, leg, and ankle injuries. Head injuries such as skull fractures are not dealt with in this chapter; they are covered in the section dealing with disorders affecting consciousness (see Head injury p.93).

Use the questionnaire on page 114 to test your understanding of first aid for bone, joint, and muscle injuries.

Contents

Dealing with a broken bone	**102**
Types of bone, joint, and muscle injury	**104**
Jaw injury	**106**
Cheek and nose injury	**106**
Collarbone injury	**107**
Arm injury	**108**
Hand and finger injury	**108**
Rib injury	**109**
Pelvic injury	**109**
Spinal injury	**110**
Leg injury	**111**
Ankle injury	**112**
Knee injury	**113**
Cramp	**113**
Test yourself	**114**

Dealing with a broken bone

Bones are normally very strong but they can break or crack if they are struck or twisted (p.104). Injuries can also occur if bones at a joint are pulled out of their normal position, if the ligaments that support the joints are torn, or if the muscles are torn (p.105). It can be difficult to distinguish between a bone, joint, or muscle injury without an X-ray or a scan, so if you are in any doubt, treat the injury as a broken bone. You need to protect the casualty from further injury or damage by keeping him as still as possible until help arrives.

WARNING
▶ Do not move the casualty unnecessarily.
▶ If it is necessary to move the casualty, enlist the help of others and plan the move before you start. Make sure the injured part is secured and supported.

Check for danger
Make sure there are no further risks to you or the casualty. Remove the ladder if it is safe to do so

Get a history
Ask the casualty what has happened. He may tell you he heard or felt a bone break

Keep casualty still
Tell the casualty to stay still and make sure he understands how important it is not to move

Watch for shock
Look for signs of shock, such as pallor and sweating. The casualty may complain of feelings of nausea, faintness, and dizziness

Pain and tenderness
The casualty may tell you that he is in great pain and that the area around the injury is tender

Swelling around injury
The affected area may appear swollen and bruised; however, this may not be evident at first

Check for deformity
The affected part of the body may appear deformed compared to the other side of the body

Give reassurance
Explain to the casualty what you are doing to help reassure him and keep him calm

What you should do

Your aims
▶ Prevent further injury
▶ Get casualty to hospital
▶ Treat any shock

IMPORTANT
▶ If the casualty is unconscious and you suspect a neck injury, use the jaw-thrust method to open the airway (p.111).

1 Support injured limb

● Leave the casualty in the position found.
● Secure and support the injured part by hand or by using rolled-up blankets or bandages depending on the site of injury.
● If the casualty has fallen from a height, suspect that he has a spinal injury and support the head and neck at all times to prevent further injury.
● Cover any wound with a sterile wound dressing or clean pad.
● Check the circulation in a limb after applying any bandages (see Roller bandages p.26).

Support head and neck to prevent movement

2 Get casualty to hospital

● The site and extent of the injury will determine how the casualty should be transported to hospital: for example, if it is an arm injury, you may be able to take him by car.
● If you suspect injury to the spine or neck, always phone for an ambulance.

3 Treat shock

● Look for signs of shock and treat the casualty accordingly (p.61).

4 Monitor casualty

● Monitor and record the casualty's vital signs – level of response, pulse, and breathing (pp.20–1) – regularly until help arrives.
● Reassure him and tell him what is happening.

IMPORTANT
▶ Do not allow the casualty to eat, drink, or smoke as a general anaesthetic may be needed later.

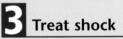
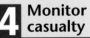

Types of bone, joint, and muscle injury

Injuries to the bones, joints, and muscles include fractures, dislocated joints, sprains, and strains. A fracture is a broken or cracked bone. A joint becomes dislocated when one of its bones is pulled out of its normal position. A sprain happens when the ligaments (the fibrous bands that hold bones together at a joint) become torn. A strain is an overstretched muscle or tendon (the fibrous band that attaches muscle to bone).

> **IMPORTANT**
> ▶ It can be difficult to tell the difference between bone, joint, and muscle injuries. Finding out how the incident happened (p.17) may indicate the type of injury to suspect. If in doubt, it is safest to treat the injury as a broken bone and seek medical help.
> ▶ Do not move the injured part of the casualty unnecessarily as you may cause further damage to blood vessels, tissues, or internal organs.
> ▶ Do not give the casualty anything to eat or drink as he may need a general anaesthetic later.

Broken bones

A considerable force is needed to break a bone unless the bone is already weakened by disease. The force can be direct, indirect, or twisting. A direct force, such as a kick, will break the bone at the point of impact. An indirect force will cause a break some distance from the point of impact; for example, a fall onto an outstretched hand may break the collarbone. A twisting force can also break a bone; this can occur when a foot that is stuck twists in a way that breaks the ankle.

Broken bones are very painful. If a large bone breaks, there will be internal bleeding from broken blood vessels in the bone. If a protective bone, such as a rib, is broken, there is a risk of damage to internal organs. Children – because their bones are still growing and flexible – may have greenstick fractures, in which a bone cracks, splits, or bends.

The injury can be stable, in which the broken ends stay in place, or unstable, in which the ends are likely to move and may break through the skin. If the ends do break through the skin, or there is a wound, the break is open. If the skin is intact, the break is closed.

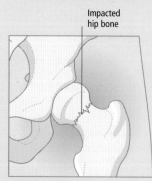

Impacted hip bone

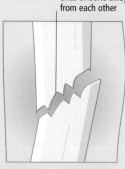

Ends of bone away from each other

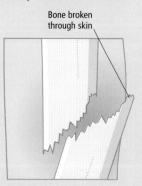

Bone broken through skin

Stable injury
In a stable injury, either the bone is not completely broken or the broken ends are impacted (wedged into each other) and the risk of further immediate damage or bleeding is small.

Unstable injury
If the broken ends of the bone can slide past each other, it is an unstable injury. Damage to the surrounding tissues and organs is possible, especially if the injured part is moved.

Open break
In an open break, the skin is broken, sometimes with the bone protruding. Bleeding is likely, and there is a risk of infection. If the skin is intact, the injury is known as a closed break.

Joint injuries

The main injuries that can affect joints are sprains and dislocations, both of which are very painful and can be slow to heal. A sprained joint generally happens when a sudden or unexpected wrenching movement stretches or tears a ligament that supports a joint. This type of injury is especially common around the ankle and may happen when a casualty twists his ankle after misjudging a step.

A dislocated joint can result from a strong force that wrenches one of the bones of a joint out of the normal position. This type of injury is most common at the shoulder, jaw, and joints in the finger or thumb – a dislocated thumb is a particularly common skiing injury. A dislocated joint in the backbone can be very serious because there may be damage to the spinal cord (p.92). In some instances, a dislocation of the shoulder or hip may damage nerves in the region of the affected joint.

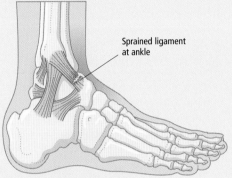

Sprained ligament at ankle

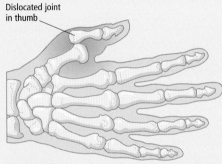

Dislocated joint in thumb

Sprained joint
When a joint is sprained, there is often swelling and bruising around the joint. The injury may also cause the joint to have a limited range of movement.

Dislocated joint
In this type of injury, the joint will appear to be misshapen, or deformed, when compared to other similar joints. There may also be swelling and bruising around the affected joint.

Muscle injuries

The muscles that move the skeleton are attached to bones by tendons. A muscle or tendon can be pulled or "strained". This type of injury often occurs at or near to the point where the muscle and tendon join to each other. A strained muscle may have just a few or many fibres torn. A strained tendon may be torn completely. These injuries are also painful.

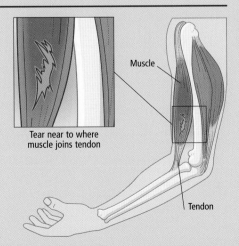

Tear near to where muscle joins tendon

Muscle

Tendon

Torn muscle and tendon
This type of injury has extensive, deep bruising, leading to severe pain and discomfort. A torn muscle or tendon usually takes a long time to heal.

Jaw injury

A broken jaw is usually caused by a direct blow to the jaw. Rarely, a blow to one side of the jaw can also fracture the other side.

SIGNS AND SYMPTOMS
▶ Pain when speaking, chewing, or swallowing
▶ Blood-stained saliva
▶ Displaced teeth
▶ Swelling and/or unevenness along jaw

Your aims	You will need
▶ Keep airway open ▶ Get casualty to hospital	▶ Soft pad

1 Keep airway open

● Lean the casualty forwards to let any fluid drain away from his mouth.
● Ask the casualty to spit out any loose teeth or dentures. Keep them to give to the doctor or ambulance crew.

2 Support jaw

● Ask the casualty to hold a soft pad loosely against his jaw.

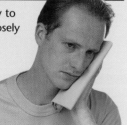

3 Get casualty to hospital

● Take or send the casualty to hospital.

WARNING
▶ If the casualty is seriously injured or is not fully conscious, put him in the recovery position (p.38 adults; p.47 children) with the injured side down and a soft pad under his head.

✚ CALL AN AMBULANCE

Cheek and nose injury

A blow of considerable force to the face, such as occurs in a car crash, is commonly the cause of a fractured cheekbone or nose.

SIGNS AND SYMPTOMS
▶ Swelling and bruising
▶ Pain around affected area

Your aims	You will need
▶ Reduce swelling ▶ Get casualty to hospital	▶ Cold compress

1 Apply cold compress

● Place a cold compress (p.25) on the injured area to reduce the swelling.

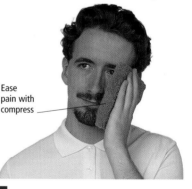

Ease pain with compress

2 Treat nosebleed

● If necessary, treat the casualty for a nosebleed (p.67).

3 Get casualty to hospital

● Take or send the casualty to hospital.

IMPORTANT
▶ If there is a yellowish, blood-stained fluid leaking from the nose, assume the casualty has a skull fracture and treat accordingly (p.93).

Collarbone injury

A broken collarbone is usually the result of indirect force, for example from falling onto an outstretched hand. This transmits force along the casualty's forearm and upper arm to the collarbone. It can also be caused by a direct blow. Collarbone injuries often occur in young people as a result of sporting activities.

Your aims	You will need
▶ Immobilise collarbone	▶ Two triangular bandages
▶ Get casualty to hospital	▶ Soft padding

SIGNS AND SYMPTOMS
▶ Pain and tenderness
▶ Casualty attempts to relieve pain by supporting the elbow and not moving the arm
▶ Swelling or deformity

1 Support arm

● Help the casualty to position her arm on the injured side so that her fingertips rest on the uninjured collarbone.
● Ask her to support the affected arm at the elbow.

Rest fingertips on collarbone

Ask casualty to support arm at elbow

2 Put arm in sling

● Put the arm in an elevation sling (p.29), being careful to move the arm as little as possible as you do so.

3 Position soft padding

● Place soft padding, such as a folded towel, between the casualty's upper arm and chest to make her more comfortable.

4 Secure arm to chest

● Secure the arm to the casualty's chest by tying a broad-fold bandage (p.27) over the sling and around her body.
● Check circulation in the thumb (see Roller bandages p.26).

Check circulation in thumb

5 Get casualty to hospital

● Take or send the casualty to hospital.

Arm injury

A break can occur anywhere along the upper arm or forearm and may involve the elbow or wrist joint.

SIGNS AND SYMPTOMS
▶ Pain and tenderness
▶ Reluctance to move injured arm
▶ Deformity, swelling, and bruising

Your aims	You will need
▶ Immobilise arm ▶ Get casualty to hospital	▶ Padding ▶ Two triangular bandages

1 Support arm

● If possible, gently bend the casualty's arm at the elbow so that her arm is positioned across her body. Ask her to support her elbow with her other hand.
● Place padding, such as a folded towel, between the site of the break and the body.

2 Put arm in sling

● Put the arm in an arm sling (p.28).
● For extra support, secure the casualty's arm to her body with a broad-fold bandage (p.27), making sure you avoid the site of the break.

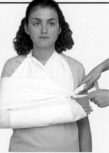

3 Get casualty to hospital

● Take or send the casualty to hospital.

WARNING
▶ If the casualty is unable to bend her arm, do not force it. Help her to lie down and place padding, such as a towel, around the injured elbow.
✚ CALL AN AMBULANCE

Hand and finger injury

Broken bones in the hands or fingers are often caused by crushing. There may also be a wound, which may cause bleeding.

SIGNS AND SYMPTOMS
▶ Pain and tenderness
▶ Reluctance to move injured hand
▶ Deformity, swelling, and bruising

Your aims	You will need
▶ Immobilise and raise injured hand ▶ Get casualty to hospital	▶ Disposable gloves ▶ Sterile wound dressing ▶ Soft padding ▶ Two triangular bandages

1 Raise hand

● If there is any bleeding, put on disposable gloves, if available. Raise the hand to control any bleeding and reduce swelling. If you can, remove any rings.

2 Support arm in sling

● If the hand or finger is bleeding, put a sterile wound dressing on it and place soft padding, such as cotton wool, around the hand.
● Support the arm in an elevation sling (p.29), securing it with a broad-fold bandage (p.27).

Support arm in elevation sling

3 Get casualty to hospital

● Take or send the casualty to hospital.

Rib injury

Broken ribs are held in place naturally because they are attached to the ribcage. To relieve the pain of a broken rib, support the arm on the affected side.

SIGNS AND SYMPTOMS
▶ Sharp pain in side, worsened by taking deep breaths, coughing, or movement
▶ Tenderness around affected ribs
▶ Crackling sound

Your aims	You will need
▶ Support casualty's chest ▶ Get casualty to hospital	▶ Two triangular bandages

1 Put arm in sling

● Make sure the casualty is in a comfortable position, preferably sitting down.
● Support the arm in an arm sling (p.28).
● If necessary, secure the arm with a broad-fold bandage (p.27).

Support arm in sling

2 Get casualty to hospital

● Take or send the casualty to hospital.

WARNING
▶ If several ribs are damaged, the casualty's breathing may be badly affected. Lean the casualty towards his injured side with his head and shoulders well supported and his knees bent.

✚ CALL AN AMBULANCE

Pelvic injury

Treat a suspected fractured pelvis with great care because there may also be injuries to organs with possible internal bleeding.

SIGNS AND SYMPTOMS
▶ Pain, swelling, and inability to walk
▶ Desire to pass urine, which may be blood-stained
▶ Possible internal bleeding and shock

Your aims	You will need
▶ Relieve shock ▶ Get casualty to hospital	▶ Padding ▶ Blanket ▶ Notepad and pen

1 Help casualty lie down

● Help the casualty onto his back with his legs straight or knees slightly bent.
● Put some padding, such as a cushion or rolled-up coat, under his knees for support.

2 Treat for shock

● If necessary, treat the casualty for shock (p.61).
● Reassure him and keep him warm.
● Do not allow him to eat or drink.

✚ CALL AN AMBULANCE

3 Monitor casualty

● Monitor and record the casualty's vital signs – level of response, pulse, and breathing (pp.20–1) – regularly until help arrives.

Spinal injury

Back injuries can be serious because they may affect the spinal cord, which contains the nerves that control many of the body's functions. A damaged spinal cord can result in paralysis of the body below the injured area. Always suspect a spinal injury if the casualty has fallen awkwardly, especially from a height, and particularly if the casualty has a head injury or is experiencing any loss of feeling or movement. Back injuries can be made worse by incorrect handling. Treat a conscious casualty as described below. For an unconscious casualty, see opposite.

Your aims	You will need
▶ Prevent further injury	▶ Coats/towels
▶ Get casualty to hospital urgently	▶ Blanket
	▶ Notepad and pen

SIGNS AND SYMPTOMS
▶ Tenderness around back
▶ Shooting pains or "electric shocks" in limbs and/or trunk
▶ Inability to feel or move legs if injury is in lower back
▶ Inability to move any limb at all if injury is at neck level

1 Keep casualty still

● Advise the casualty not to move.
● Kneeling behind the casualty's head, place your hands on either side of the head to support it with the head, neck, and spine aligned.

Leave a gap between fingers and thumb so that casualty can hear you

2 Support head, neck, and shoulders

● Use rolled-up coats or towels to protect and support the casualty's head, neck, and shoulders.
● Cover the casualty with a blanket.

✚ **CALL AN AMBULANCE**

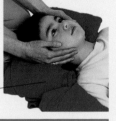

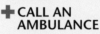

Place rolled towels around head and shoulders

IMPORTANT
▶ Do not move the casualty unless you believe his life is in danger.

For an unconscious casualty

● Kneel behind the casualty's head and place your hands on either side of the head to support it with the head, neck, and spine aligned.

● If necessary, open the casualty's airway using the jaw-thrust method. Position your hands on either side of his face with your fingertips at the angles of his jaw. Gently lift his jaw forwards with your fingers, making sure you do not tilt his head back.

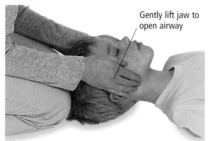

Gently lift jaw to open airway

● Check the casualty's breathing (p.37 adults; p.46 children; p.50 infants). If he is breathing, continue to support his head.

● Ask a helper to
✚ **CALL AN AMBULANCE**

● If you need to leave the casualty to call an ambulance yourself or you are unable to keep the casualty's airway open using the jaw thrust, put him into the recovery position (p.38 adults; p.47 children; p.51 infants), keeping his head and trunk aligned at all times.

● If the casualty is not breathing, begin resuscitation (pp.36–52).

● Monitor and record the casualty's vital signs – level of response, pulse, and breathing (pp.20–1) – regularly until help arrives.

Leg injury

A broken leg is a serious injury. The thighbone has a rich blood supply and a break can cause severe internal bleeding. The shinbone lies just below the skin and, if broken, it may stick through the skin (p.104), making it susceptible to infection.

SIGNS AND SYMPTOMS
▶ Pain, swelling, and loss of movement
▶ Shock may develop
▶ Open wound with broken bone visible
▶ Injured leg may appear shortened
▶ Foot, and possibly knee, turned sideways

Your aims	You will need
▶ Support injured leg ▶ Get casualty to hospital urgently	▶ Sterile wound dressing

1 Support leg

● Help the casualty to lie down carefully.
● Gently steady and support the leg with your hands at the joints above and below the site of the break.

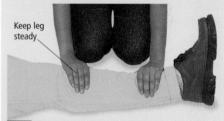

Keep leg steady

2 Treat wounds

● Cover any wounds with a sterile wound dressing (p.24).
✚ **CALL AN AMBULANCE**

3 Treat for shock

● Continue to support the leg to prevent any movement until the ambulance arrives. If necessary, treat for shock (p.61).

Ankle injury

A sprained ankle is the result of the ligaments that hold the bones together at the joints becoming stretched or torn (p.105). This injury is usually very painful and the symptoms can easily be mistaken for a broken bone (p.104). An ankle strain occurs when the muscles and tendons are torn by a sudden movement or violent contraction. Both injuries frequently take place during sporting activities.

Your aims	You will need
▶ Reduce swelling and pain	▶ Cold compress
▶ Get casualty to hospital if necessary or seek medical help	▶ Cotton-wool padding
	▶ Roller bandage

SIGNS AND SYMPTOMS
▶ Swelling
▶ Pain and tenderness
▶ Inability to move ankle or stand on affected limb
▶ Gradual bruising

IMPORTANT
▶ Follow the RICE procedure if you suspect the casualty has a sprain or a strain:

R	I	C	E
Rest	Ice	Compress	Elevate

▶ If you suspect the casualty has a serious injury, for example he is in great pain and unable to move the affected foot,

✚ **TAKE OR SEND CASUALTY TO HOSPITAL**

1 Apply cold compress

● Help the casualty to sit or lie down.
● Support the ankle in a comfortable position, such as on your knee.
● If the injury has just occurred, cool the ankle by applying a cold compress (p.25) for 10 minutes and then reassess the injury. Reapply a cold compress at 10-minute intervals for up to 30 minutes if necessary.

Reduce swelling with a compress

2 Bandage around ankle

● Place cotton-wool padding against the ankle and press gently.
● Secure the padding with a roller bandage, leaving the toes exposed (p.26).
● Check the circulation in the toes (p.26) every 10 minutes.

Bandage around padding

3 Raise limb

● Raise and support the injured limb to reduce the flow of blood to the injury, thereby reducing bruising.
● If the injury appears to be minor, advise the casualty to rest and to seek medical help, if necessary.

Knee injury

It can be difficult to tell whether a person has a broken kneecap or has damaged cartilage or a ligament. If you are in any doubt, treat the injury as described below. The knee-cap can be broken by a direct blow or split by a violent pull from the thigh muscles attached to it.

SIGNS AND SYMPTOMS
▶ Extreme pain
▶ Swelling

Your aim	You will need
▶ Get casualty to hospital urgently	▶ Pillows/coats ▶ Cotton-wool roll ▶ Roller bandage

1 Support leg

● Help the casualty to lie down.
● Steady and support her leg in a comfortable position.
● Place padding such as a pillow under her knee and rolled coats and/or pillows around her leg.

2 Bandage knee

● Wrap soft padding such as cotton wool around the knee.
● Secure the soft padding gently with a roller bandage (p.26).

✚ CALL AN AMBULANCE

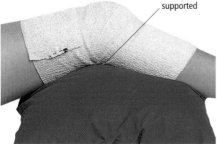

Keep leg steady and supported

Cramp

This pain can occur suddenly and is usually caused by a tightening, or contraction, of a single muscle or a group of muscles. Cramp can normally be relieved by stretching the affected muscles.

Your aim
▶ Relieve pain

In the hand

● Straighten the casualty's bent fingers by gently stretching them backwards.
● Massage the hand to relieve the cramp still further.

In the foot

● Straighten the casualty's bent toes by gently pushing them upwards.
● Help the casualty to stand on the ball of her foot.

In the calf

● Straighten the casualty's knee and pull the foot up towards the shin as far as possible.
● Gently massage the calf muscles.

Raise affected leg

In the back of the thigh

● Straighten the casualty's knee by pulling the leg up and forwards, and gently but firmly press the knee down.

IMPORTANT
▶ Cramp may occur if a person has been sweating heavily. To relieve this, give the casualty plenty of water to drink.

Test yourself

Now that you have read and studied the chapter on first-aid treatments for bone, joint, and muscle injuries, see if you can answer the questions below. Check your answers against the correct ones on page 144.

1 Which of the following should be your priorities when looking after a casualty with a broken leg?
  a Immobilise the leg............................☐
  b Reduce the swelling by cooling with water ....☐
  c Encourage the casualty to try standing on the leg....................☐
  d Watch for shock...............................☐

2 What is an open break?
....
....

3 What is the risk with an open break that is not present with a closed break?
....
....

4 If you suspect that a casualty has a broken bone, why should you not give him anything to eat, drink, or smoke?
....
....

5 What is the difference between a sprain and a strain?
....
....
....
....

6 How is a collarbone usually broken?
....
....

7 What are the signs and symptoms that might make you suspect that a casualty's forearm is broken?
....
....
....

8 What are the likely complications if a casualty has a pelvic injury?
....
....

9 What is your most important priority when dealing with a casualty who has a suspected broken bone?
....
....
....

10 What do the letters R I C E stand for?
R ....
I ....
C ....
E ....

11 For how long should you leave a cold compress on an ankle injury?
....
....
....
....

12 How would you relieve cramp in a calf muscle?
....
....

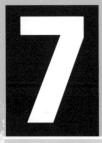

Poisoning, bites, and stings

This chapter begins by explaining what to do if you suspect that someone has swallowed a poison. The effects of a poison vary considerably depending on what it is and how much is consumed. Poisoning is usually non-intentional and can be caused by exposure to toxic substances or eating or drinking them. It can also be caused by alcohol or drugs.

First-aid treatments for insect stings, which can be serious if a casualty is allergic to the sting, and snake bites, which require prompt attention to prevent venom (poison) from spreading around the body, are also covered. Finally, the chapter sets out how to deal with animal bites, which always require medical attention because they may carry a risk of rabies and tetanus infections.

Use the questionnaire on page 122 to test your understanding of first aid for poisoning, bites, and stings.

Contents

Dealing with poisoning	116
Alcohol and drug poisoning	118
Insect stings	119
Snake bites	120
Animal bites	121
Marine injuries	121
Test yourself	122

Dealing with poisoning

Poisons are substances that can cause temporary or permanent damage to the body if taken in large enough quantities. Poisons can be swallowed, absorbed or injected through the skin, splashed into the eyes, or breathed in through the lungs. The effects vary according to the poison and how it has been taken. Try to find out what was taken and how much – if the casualty is conscious, ask what happened as soon as possible, in case she loses consciousness. If there are bystanders, ask them.

Check for danger
Make sure there are no risks to you or the casualty

Monitor level of consciousness
Depending on the poison and the quantity taken, the casualty may be unconscious or may lose consciousness at any time

Give reassurance
Talk to the casualty to reassure her and keep her calm

Look for burns around mouth
If a corrosive substance has been swallowed, the lips may look burnt and feel painful

Check breathing
Note whether the casualty's breathing is noisy, difficult, or normal

Upset stomach
If the casualty has swallowed a poison, she may vomit or, at a later stage, have diarrhoea

WARNING

▶ If the casualty becomes unconscious, be ready to begin resuscitation if necessary (pp.36–52).

▶ If you need to give rescue breaths and there are chemicals around the casualty's mouth, use either a face shield or the mouth-to-nose method to protect yourself.

What you should do

Your aims

▶ Identify poison
▶ Get casualty to hospital urgently
▶ Monitor casualty

IMPORTANT

▶ Take care not to get any of the chemical on yourself. If you do, wash it off (see Chemical burns p.81).

▶ Do not leave the casualty alone unless you have to do so to call an ambulance.

1 Identify poison

● Look for any evidence of what the casualty has taken: for example berries, medicine bottles, or pills.

2 Call an ambulance

● Phone for an ambulance.
● Give details of the poison involved and the amount the casualty has taken.
● Keep any evidence of the poison taken for the ambulance personnel.
● If the casualty vomits, keep a sample for the ambulance personnel.

3 Treat corrosive poison

● If the poison has burned the casualty's lips, give her sips of water or milk to help cool them.
● Do not try to make the casualty vomit. If she has taken a corrosive substance that burns going to her stomach, it will burn again coming up.

4 Monitor casualty

● Monitor and record the casualty's vital signs – level of response, pulse, and breathing (pp.20–1) – regularly until help arrives.
● Watch especially for any deterioration in the level of response.
● Pass on this information to the emergency services.

Get a history
Ask the casualty what she has taken. Look for clues nearby, such as containers, to identify the poison

Give details of poison to emergency services

Alcohol and drug poisoning

Taken in excess, alcohol and drugs can seriously affect all physical and mental abilities. This can result in a casualty falling and sustaining other injuries. If the casualty is not fully conscious, there is a risk that he may vomit and inhale the vomit. Since alcohol and some drugs dilate the skin's blood vessels, the casualty will lose heat and may develop hypothermia (p.86). If a casualty smells of alcohol, excess alcohol may not be the only problem; check for other health problems, such as a stroke (p.96) or a heart attack (p.124).

Your aims	You will need
▶ Keep casualty warm	▶ Blanket/coat
▶ Check for other injuries and illnesses	▶ Notepad and pen
▶ Get medical help if necessary	

SIGNS AND SYMPTOMS
▶ Smell of alcohol
▶ Loss of coordination; confusion
▶ Flushed face
▶ Deep, noisy breathing

If casualty becomes unconscious:
▶ Shallow breathing and weak pulse

If stimulant drugs have been taken:
▶ Raised body temperature and other symptoms of heatstroke (p.85)

1 Cover casualty

● Help the casualty to sit or lie down in a warm, comfortable place if possible.
● Cover him with a blanket or coat to help keep him warm.

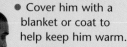

Put a blanket or coat over casualty

2 Look for causes

● Look for empty containers that may indicate what the casualty has taken.
● Keep a sample of any vomit in case it needs to be analysed.
● Treat any injuries.

3 Monitor casualty

● Get medical help if necessary.
● Monitor and record his vital signs (pp.20–1) regularly until help arrives.

Use of stimulant drugs

Stimulant drugs, such as ecstasy and cocaine, can lead to excitable, hyperactive behaviour and possibly hallucinations, exhaustion, and overheating. For a casualty needing first aid after taking a stimulant drug:
● Lower his body temperature by getting him to rest in a cool place (see Heatstroke p.85).
● Do not cover him with a blanket as this will increase his body temperature.

WARNING
▶ If the casualty is unconscious, open the airway and check breathing. Put him in the recovery position if he is breathing. Be ready to begin resuscitation (pp.36–52).

✚ CALL AN AMBULANCE

Insect stings

The stings of a bee, wasp, or hornet are usually more alarming than dangerous, although multiple stings and stings in the mouth can be serious (below). Some people are allergic to stings (see Anaphylactic shock p.129) and will need urgent medical help.

Your aims	You will need
▶ Remove sting	▶ Rigid piece of plastic, such as a credit card, to scrape off sting
▶ Relieve pain and swelling	
▶ Get medical help if necessary	▶ Ice pack
	For stings in mouth or throat:
	▶ Ice cubes/cold water

SIGNS AND SYMPTOMS
▶ Pain at site of sting
▶ Slightly swollen, red, and sore skin

WARNING
▶ If the casualty shows any signs of anaphylactic shock (p.129),
✚ **CALL AN AMBULANCE**

1 Remove sting

● If you can see the sting, scrape it away carefully with your fingernail or a credit card.

Use credit card to scrape sting away

IMPORTANT
▶ Do not try to remove an insect sting with tweezers because the sting may have a venom sac attached and you may squeeze more venom into the casualty.

2 Apply ice pack

● Place an ice pack (p.25) on the affected area to reduce pain and swelling.

3 Rest injured part

● Keep the injured part in a comfortable position, preferably raised, until the pain and swelling ease.
● If you are concerned about continued pain and swelling,
✚ **GET MEDICAL HELP**

Stings in the mouth or throat

● A sting inside the mouth or throat is potentially very dangerous because the swelling it causes can obstruct the casualty's airway. If you suspect a mouth or throat sting,

✚ **CALL AN AMBULANCE**

● If possible, give the casualty an ice cube to suck or sips of cold water to reduce the swelling of the tissues lining the airway.

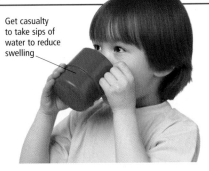

Get casualty to take sips of water to reduce swelling

Snake bites

The adder is the only venomous snake native to the British Isles, although exotic venomous snakes are often kept as pets. To prevent snake venom spreading through the body, keep the casualty still and make sure the heart is above the level of the wound.

Your aims	You will need
▶ Stop venom spreading through body	▶ Soap and water
▶ Reassure casualty	▶ Clean gauze swabs or other non-fluffy material
▶ Get casualty to hospital urgently	▶ Crepe roller bandage
	▶ Towels/blanket
	▶ Triangular bandage

SIGNS AND SYMPTOMS
▶ One or two small puncture marks
▶ Pain, redness, and possible swelling
▶ Nausea and vomiting
▶ Disturbed vision
▶ Sweating

WARNING
▶ Do not try to suck out the venom.
▶ If the casualty becomes unconscious, open the airway and check breathing. Put her in the recovery position if she is breathing. Be ready to begin resuscitation if necessary (pp.36–52).

1 Help casualty lie down

● Help the casualty to lie down and tell her to keep still to slow down the spread of venom in the body.
● Reassure her.

2 Call an ambulance

● Phone for an ambulance. If you can, describe the snake so the hospital knows which antivenom to give the casualty.

3 Clean wound

● If possible, wash around the wound with soap and water.
● Pat the area dry with clean gauze swabs or other non-fluffy material.
● Wrap a crepe roller bandage around the limb above the wound. Do not cover the bite.

4 Keep injured part still

● Place padding, such as rolled-up towels or blankets, around the injured area. Keep the padding in place with a triangular bandage (p.27).
● If a leg has been bitten, tie both legs together with triangular bandages.

Keep heart above level of bite to minimise spread of venom

Secure padding around injured limb to keep it still

Leave bite exposed

Animal bites

Sharp teeth make deep wounds so animal bites can be serious. Prompt first aid is needed if the skin is broken to prevent infection. Animal bites carry the risk of tetanus infection or, more seriously, rabies, especially if the bite occurred overseas.

Your aims	You will need
▶ Control bleeding	▶ Disposable gloves
▶ Prevent infection	▶ Soap and water
▶ Get medical help if necessary	▶ Clean gauze swabs
	▶ Plaster or sterile wound dressing

IMPORTANT
▶ If there is a possibility of rabies, take or send the casualty to hospital immediately.
▶ Seek medical help if the casualty has never had a tetanus injection, does not know when he was last injected or how many injections he has had, or it is more than 10 years since his last tetanus injection (p.62).

1 Press on wound

● Put on disposable gloves if available.
● If the wound is bleeding, press on the wound and raise the limb.

2 Clean and cover wound

● Wash the wound thoroughly with soap and water.
● Pat the wound dry with clean gauze swabs.
● Cover the wound with a plaster or sterile wound dressing.

3 Get medical help

● If the wound is large or deep, take or send the casualty to hospital.

Marine injuries

Certain marine animals, such as corals and sea anemones, have painful stings that can be relieved with an ice pack. More serious injuries can be caused by tropical jellyfish stings and embedded spines from animals such as sea urchins and weever fish.

Your aims	You will need
▶ Reduce swelling	▶ Ice pack
▶ Get casualty to hospital if necessary	For a tropical jellyfish sting:
	▶ Vinegar or sea water
	▶ Roller bandage
	For an embedded spine:
	▶ Hot water

1 Help casualty sit or lie down

● Get the casualty to sit or lie down.
● Reassure the casualty.

2 Apply ice pack

● Place an ice pack (p.25) on the affected area for 10 minutes.

IMPORTANT
▶ If the injury is severe or if the casualty suffers a serious reaction to the sting,
✚ CALL AN AMBULANCE

For a tropical jellyfish sting

● Pour lots of vinegar or sea water over the wound.
● Lightly cover the wound with a roller bandage.
✚ CALL AN AMBULANCE

For an embedded spine

● Soak the injured part in water as hot as the casualty can bear to relieve pain.
● Take or send the casualty to hospital to have the spine removed.

Test yourself

Now that you have read and studied the chapter on first-aid treatments for poisoning, bites, and stings, see if you can answer the questions below. Check your answers against the correct ones on page 144.

1 What are your aims when dealing with poisoning?

....
....
....

2 If you need to give rescue breaths to an unconscious poisoned casualty who has chemicals around his mouth, what should you do?

....
....

3 Which of the following are signs or symptoms of alcohol poisoning?
  a Smell of alcohol on casualty ....☐
  b Loss of coordination..........................☐
  c Confusion......................................☐
  d Flushed face...................................☐
  e Deep, noisy breathing.......................☐
  f Loss of consciousness........................☐

4 Why should you keep a casualty with alcohol poisoning warm?

....
....

5 What is your priority when dealing with a casualty who has taken stimulant drugs?

....
....

6 What is the best way to remove an insect sting?

....
....

7 Why should you not use tweezers to remove an insect sting?

....
....

8 Why is an insect sting in the mouth or throat particularly dangerous?

....
....

9 List three things to do to stop the spread of snake venom after a bite.
1...
2...
3...

10 What infections do animal bites carry the risk of?

....
....

11 What first aid would you give for a sea anemone sting?

....
....
....

12 What first aid would you give for a tropical jellyfish sting?

....
....
....

8 Medical problems and emergencies

This chapter covers a wide range of medical problems and emergencies that can affect a casualty. It begins by explaining how to deal with someone who is having a heart attack. This is a life-threatening condition and every first aider needs to be aware of the risk that the heart may stop beating.

There are first-aid procedures for serious disorders that require urgent medical help, such as a diabetic emergency and anaphylactic shock. However, this chapter also deals with minor illnesses and disorders, such as headache, sore throat, and fever. While these are usually no cause for concern, it is important to be aware that they can be symptoms of a serious illness, such as meningitis.

Use the questionnaire on page 139 to test your understanding of first aid for medical problems and emergencies.

Contents

Dealing with a heart attack	124
Angina	126
Diabetic emergency	127
Allergy	128
Anaphylactic shock	129
Asthma	130
Croup	131
Object in the eye	132
Object in the ear	133
Object in the nose	133
Toothache	134
Earache	134
Headache	135
Migraine	135
Sore throat	136
Fever	136
Meningitis	137
Abdominal pain	138
Vomiting and diarrhoea	138
Test yourself	139

Dealing with a heart attack

A heart attack is caused by a blockage, usually a blood clot, that forms in an artery carrying blood to part of the heart muscle. This blockage is known as coronary thrombosis and its effects depend on how much of the heart muscle is damaged. The main risk of a heart attack is that the heart will go into an abnormal rhythm – ventricular fibrillation – and stop beating (cardiac arrest). If you suspect a heart attack, encourage the casualty to rest and arrange for him to be taken to hospital as soon as possible.

Get a history
Ask the casualty or a bystander what has happened and whether the casualty has any history of heart problems or angina

Check for signs
Look at the casualty – he may appear ashen, sweaty, and blue around the lips

Check for symptoms
Ask the casualty how he is feeling. He may complain of breathlessness, nausea, dizziness, and a sense that he is seriously ill

Pain in chest
Ask the casualty if he is in pain – he will usually feel a crushing pain in his chest that may radiate into his arms or jaw

Loss of consciousness
The casualty's heartbeat and breathing may stop suddenly. Be ready to begin resuscitation if necessary

Help casualty rest
Make him as comfortable as possible; sit him down so that his head and shoulders are supported and his knees bent

Give reassurance
Tell the casualty that you will call an ambulance and help him to take any medication

What you should do

Your aims
▶ Encourage casualty to rest
▶ Get casualty to hospital urgently

IMPORTANT
▶ Do not leave the casualty alone unless you have to do so in order to get help.
▶ Do not allow the casualty to eat, drink, or smoke.

1 Help casualty sit down

● Help the casualty to sit down, making him as comfortable as possible.
● Ideally, help him lean back against a wall or chair so that his head and shoulders are supported and his knees are bent.

2 Call an ambulance

● Phone for an ambulance immediately.
● Tell the operator that you suspect the casualty has had a heart attack.

3 Give aspirin

● If the casualty is conscious, give him a 300 mg aspirin tablet to chew slowly.

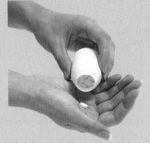

4 Give any other medication

● If the casualty has any other medication, such as an aerosol for angina, help him to take it.

5 Regularly check casualty

● Monitor and record the casualty's vital signs – level of response, pulse, and breathing (pp.20–1) – regularly until help arrives. Watch for deterioration.

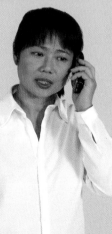

Angina

A person with angina feels a tight pain in the chest due to a narrowing of the arteries, resulting in an inadequate supply of oxygen and nutrients to the heart muscle. It is usually brought on by exercise and relieved by rest, but it may also be caused by anything that increases the activity of the heart, such as extreme emotion or excitement.

Your aims	You will need
▶ Help casualty to rest to ease strain on heart ▶ Help casualty take his own medication ▶ Get medical help if necessary	▶ Casualty's own medication

SIGNS AND SYMPTOMS
▶ Pain in middle of chest, sometimes spreading to jaw or arms
▶ Pain that eases with rest
▶ Breathlessness
▶ Anxiety

1 Get casualty to rest

● Help the casualty to sit down.
● Make sure he feels comfortable.
● Reassure him.

2 Help casualty take medication

● If necessary, help the casualty to find his medication.
● Help him to correctly identify his medication.
● Help him to take his medication.

3 Get medical help

● Advise the casualty to seek medical help if he is still anxious after the angina has has gone away.

Help casualty to rest and reassure him

WARNING
▶ If the pain does not ease after the casualty has rested and taken medication or if the angina returns, suspect a heart attack and

✚ CALL AN AMBULANCE

▶ Treat as for a heart attack (p.124) and be ready to begin resuscitation if necessary (pp.36–52).
▶ If the casualty becomes unconscious, open the airway and check breathing. Put him in the recovery position if he is breathing. Be ready to begin resuscitation if necessary (pp.36–52).

Diabetic emergency

A person who is diabetic is unable to produce the right amounts of insulin in the body, a chemical that controls how much sugar there is in the blood. Too much insulin results in abnormally low levels of sugar in the blood, a condition known as hypoglycaemia. Too little insulin leads to a build-up of sugar in the blood, a condition known as hyperglycaemia. Both conditions can be serious.

Hypoglycaemia

Your aims	You will need
▶ Increase sugar content in blood ▶ Get medical help	▶ Sugary drink or sweet food ▶ Notepad and pen

SIGNS AND SYMPTOMS
- ▶ Medic-Alert bracelet/syringe/tablets or gel
- ▶ Sweating; cold, clammy, and pale skin
- ▶ Strong pulse and heart palpitations
- ▶ Hunger, weakness, and faintness
- ▶ Confusion and low level of response
- ▶ Shallow breathing

1 Give sugary drink or food

- ● Help the casualty to sit down. Give him a sugary drink or something sweet to eat.

2 Advise casualty to rest

- ● If the casualty starts to feel better, give him more food or drink.
- ● Advise him to rest and to see his doctor as soon as possible.

Hyperglycaemia

Your aim	You will need
▶ Get casualty to hospital urgently	▶ Notepad and pen

SIGNS AND SYMPTOMS
- ▶ Dry skin
- ▶ Deep, heavy breathing; fast pulse
- ▶ Breath smelling of acetone (acetone smells like nail varnish remover or pear drops)
- ▶ Extreme thirst
- ▶ Casualty may become dazed and confused and may eventually lose consciousness

1 Call an ambulance

- ● If you suspect that the casualty is suffering from hyperglycaemia, phone for an ambulance immediately.

2 Monitor casualty

- ● Monitor and record his vital signs – level of response, breathing, and pulse (pp.20–1) – regularly until help arrives.

IMPORTANT
▶ It can be difficult to tell whether a casualty is suffering from hypoglycaemia or hyperglycaemia. If the casualty appears unwell and you know that he is diabetic, give him something sugary to drink. This will quickly correct hypoglycaemia and cause little harm if he is suffering from hyperglycaemia.

For an unconscious casualty with hypo- or hyperglycaemia

- ● Open the casualty's airway and check breathing. Put him in the recovery position if he is breathing. Be ready to begin resuscitation if necessary (pp.36–52).

✚ **CALL AN AMBULANCE**
- ● Monitor and record the casualty's vital signs – level of response, breathing, and pulse (pp.20–1) – regularly until help arrives.

Allergy

An allergy occurs when the body reacts to a substance, such as a food, chemical, drug, or plant pollen, that for most people is usually harmless. Symptoms of an allergy vary depending on the substance that triggers it. The most common ones include breathing difficulties, such as asthma (p.130), skin rashes, abdominal pain (p.138), or vomiting and diarrhoea (p.138). Some people may experience very severe allergic reactions that can be life-threatening (see Anaphylactic shock opposite).

Your aims	You will need
▶ Check severity of allergy	▶ Drinking water
▶ Treat mild symptoms	▶ Casualty's own medication
▶ Get medical help	

SIGNS AND SYMPTOMS
- ▶ Itchy red rash or raised areas of skin
- ▶ Breathing difficulties
- ▶ Abdominal pain
- ▶ Vomiting and diarrhoea

1 Check symptoms

- ● Find out how severe the casualty's symptoms are.
- ● Ask her if she has any known allergies.

2 Treat mild symptoms

- ● If the casualty has vomited, give her water to sip.
- ● Make her comfortable.
- ● Help the casualty take any medication that she might already have for her allergy.

3 Get medical help

- ● Advise casualty to seek medical help.

Give casualty drink to sip

Help casualty take prescribed allergy medication

IMPORTANT
▶ If the allergic reaction worsens, ask the casualty if she has any medication, such as an auto-injector, to treat anaphylactic shock (opposite). Be prepared to help her use the auto-injector.

▶ If you are still concerned about the casualty's condition or if she finds it difficult to breathe or appears distressed,

✚ **CALL AN AMBULANCE**

Anaphylactic shock

This is a severe allergic reaction that may occur after an insect sting or after eating certain foods, such as peanuts. The reaction can be fast; the casualty may find it hard to breathe and will need urgent medical help as she may lose consciousness. Some people know they suffer from this condition and carry epinephrine (adrenaline) with them – often in the form of a pre-loaded syringe called an auto-injector. Help the casualty to administer the medication or, if you are trained to do so, administer it yourself.

Your aim
▶ Get casualty to hospital urgently

1 Call an ambulance

● Phone for an ambulance immediately.

2 Ease breathing

● Help the casualty into a sitting position to ease any breathing difficulties.
● Help her to find and use any prescribed medication, such as an auto-injector.
● If the casualty is unable to use her auto-injector and you have been trained in its use, give it to her yourself.

Casualty may have difficulty breathing

Remain calm and reassure casualty

3 Provide information

● Give the ambulance crew any information that will help identify the cause of the anaphylactic reaction.

SIGNS AND SYMPTOMS
▶ Anxiety
▶ Breathing difficulties and wheezing
▶ Blotchy, red skin
▶ Swollen face and neck; puffy eyes
▶ Fast pulse

WARNING
▶ If the casualty becomes unconscious, open the airway and check breathing. Put her in the recovery position if she is breathing. Be ready to begin resuscitation if necessary (pp.36–52).

Using auto-injectors

A casualty with a known allergy may have her own medication to take in case of an attack. This usually takes the form of a syringe or auto-injector of epinephrine (adrenaline).
To give it to her:
• Hold the injector with your fingers and remove the protective cap.
• Holding the injector with your fist, place the tip firmly against the casualty's thigh to release the medication. Rub the injection site.

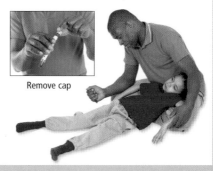

Remove cap

Asthma

An asthma attack occurs when a person's airways narrow, causing wheezing and breathing difficulties. A stimulus, such as dust, can trigger an attack or asthma may occur for no apparent reason. Most asthmatics use a reliever inhaler to treat themselves. Reassuring the casualty may help to make him feel less anxious and ease an attack.

Your aims
▶ Help casualty breathe more easily
▶ Get medical help if necessary

1 Reassure casualty

● Remain calm and reassure the casualty.
● Help him to find and use a reliever inhaler, if he has one; using it should help him to breathe more easily. Tell him to try to breathe slowly and deeply.

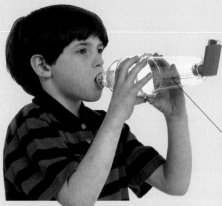

Use a reliever inhaler to make breathing easier

2 Make casualty comfortable

● Help the casualty to relax in the position that he finds most comfortable – this will usually be sitting slightly forwards with the arms resting on a firm surface, such as the back of a chair.
● If the attack has not passed within 3 minutes, ask the casualty to take another dose of his inhaler.
● If you are concerned, advise the casualty to seek medical advice.

SIGNS AND SYMPTOMS
▶ Difficulty breathing, especially breathing out
▶ Wheezy cough
▶ Anxiety and signs of distress
▶ Bluish tinge to lips and face
▶ Tiredness
▶ Difficulty talking

3 Call an ambulance

● It is necessary to phone for an ambulance if the attack is severe and the casualty has difficulty talking; if his breathing has not improved 5 minutes after using the inhaler; if he is becoming exhausted; or if this is his first attack.
● Help the casualty to use his inhaler every 5–10 minutes while you wait for the ambulance and continue to reassure him.

IMPORTANT
▶ Do not force a casualty to lie down during an asthma attack.
▶ Do not ask the casualty unnecessary questions; answering you will make him even more breathless.

WARNING
▶ If the casualty loses consciousness, open the airway and check breathing. Put him in the recovery position if he is breathing. Be ready to begin resuscitation if necessary (pp.36–52).
▶ Monitor and record the casualty's vital signs – level of response, pulse, and breathing (pp.20–1) – regularly until help arrives.

Croup

An attack of croup is caused when a young child's larynx and windpipe (trachea) become inflamed, making breathing difficult. The noise a child with croup makes may sound alarming, but the symptoms will usually pass quickly without causing the child any lasting damage. A child is more likely to suffer an attack of croup at night.

Your aims
▶ Comfort and support child
▶ Make breathing easier

SIGNS AND SYMPTOMS
▶ Distressed breathing
▶ Short, barking cough
▶ Whistling noise, especially when child breathes in
▶ Blue-grey skin (cyanosis) in severe cases

1 Comfort child

● Sit the child on your knee, make him feel secure, and reassure him.

2 Make steamy atmosphere

● To ease breathing, create a steamy atmosphere either in the bathroom by running the hot water tap in the bath or in the kitchen by boiling the kettle.
● Encourage the child to breathe in the steam.
● After his breathing eases, put the child back to bed.
● Create a steamy atmosphere in the bedroom, if possible, perhaps by hanging a wet towel over a hot radiator.

IMPORTANT
▶ If the croup is severe, persists, or you are worried,
✚ **CALL AN AMBULANCE**

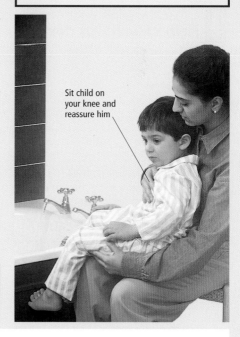

Sit child on your knee and reassure him

Epiglottitis

This disorder is caused by the epiglottis – the small, flap-like structure in the back of the throat – becoming inflamed. It is a life-threatening condition because the swollen epiglottis may block the airway. It can affect children and adults.

The signs and symptoms of epiglottitis are:
● High temperature
● Distressed breathing
● Difficulty coughing
● Difficulty swallowing
● Whistling noise when breathing in and out
● The casualty is obviously ill but sits upright.

If you suspect epiglottitis,
✚ **CALL AN AMBULANCE**
● Do not try to ease the breathing by putting your fingers down the throat; this may cause the muscles in the throat to go into spasm and quickly block the airway.

Object in the eye

The most common types of foreign object that get into the eyes are pieces of grit, dust, eyelashes, or small insects. Most of them are quite easily removed. However, you should not attempt to remove anything that sticks to the eye because this may cause damage.

Your aims	You will need
▶ Prevent injury to eye ▶ Remove foreign object	▶ Jug of water or sterile eyewash ▶ Bowl and towel ▶ Moist gauze pad/ clean handkerchief

SIGNS AND SYMPTOMS
▶ Pain or discomfort in eye; blurred vision
▶ Redness and watering of the eye

1 Help casualty sit down

● Tell the casualty not to rub her eye.
● Ask her to sit down in a chair facing a light and to lean back slightly.

2 Examine eye

● Stand behind the casualty and ask her to look up.
● Supporting her chin, gently separate the eyelids and look for the foreign object.

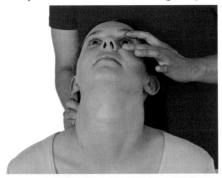

IMPORTANT
▶ Do not remove anything from the coloured part of the eye or anything that is stuck in the eye. Instead, cover the eye with a sterile wound dressing and get the casualty to hospital.

WARNING
▶ If you are unable to remove the foreign object,
✚ **TAKE OR SEND CASUALTY TO HOSPITAL**

3 Removing an object on eyelid or white of eye

● If you can see the object inside the eyelid or on the white of the eye, pour water or sterile eyewash into the inner corner of the eye to flush it out. Place a towel on the casualty's shoulder and get her to hold a bowl to catch any drips.
● If this does not work, lift it off with a moist gauze pad or clean handkerchief.

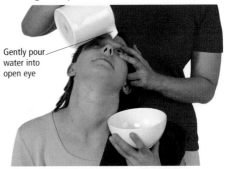

Gently pour water into open eye

4 Removing an object under upper eyelid

● If the particle is under the upper lid, ask the casualty to look down, grasp her upper lid by the lashes, and draw it out and down over the lower lid.
● If the object is still there, bathe the eye with water or eyewash and ask her to blink; the object should float off.

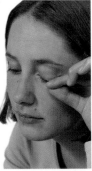

Object in the ear

Young children have a habit of putting objects such as beads into their ears; adults may leave cotton wool in theirs after cleaning them; and insects may fly or crawl into ears. A foreign object in the ear may cause temporary deafness or even damage the eardrum.

Your aims	You will need
▶ Reassure casualty	For removing an insect:
▶ Prevent injury to ear	▶ Towel
▶ Remove foreign object	▶ Tepid water
	▶ Jug/glass

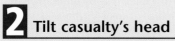 Examine ear

● Reassure the casualty.
● Look into the ear to see what the foreign object is.

2 Tilt casualty's head

● If the object is a bead or something similar, tilt the casualty's head so that the affected ear is facing downwards; the object may drop out.

> **WARNING**
> ▶ If the object does not fall out of the ear, do not try to dig it out with your fingers or any other instrument.
> ✚ **TAKE OR SEND CASUALTY TO HOSPITAL**

Removing an insect

● If an insect is in the casualty's ear, tell her to tilt her head to one side with the affected ear facing up.
● Place a towel over her shoulder and support her head with your hand.
● Gently pour tepid water from a jug or glass into the ear; the insect should float to the surface.
● If the insect does not float to the surface, get the casualty to hospital.

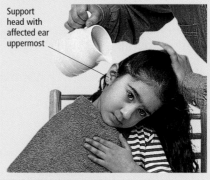

Support head with affected ear uppermost

Object in the nose

It is quite common for young children to push small objects up their noses. These may block the nose and cause an infection. If the object is sharp, it may damage the lining of the nose.

1 Reassure casualty

● Try to keep the casualty quiet and calm; tell him to breathe steadily through the mouth.
● Do not try to remove the foreign object, even if you can see it.

Your aims
▶ Reassure casualty
▶ Get casualty to hospital

SIGNS AND SYMPTOMS
▶ Difficult or noisy breathing through nose
▶ Swelling of nose
▶ Smelly or bloodstained discharge from nose

2 Get casualty to hospital

● Take or send the casualty to hospital.

Toothache

Decay in a tooth is usually the cause of toothache, especially if the pain does not go away. Toothache is often made worse by hot or cold food or drink. If it is a throbbing pain, there may be an infection at the root of the tooth.

Your aims	You will need
▶ Relieve pain	▶ Hot-water bottle
▶ Advise casualty to see a dentist	▶ Towel
	▶ Cotton wool
	▶ Oil of cloves

1 Relieve pain

● An adult may take two paracetamol tablets and a child may be given the recommended dose of paracetamol syrup.
● Give the casualty a hot-water bottle wrapped in a towel to hold against his cheek. Alternatively, give him a rolled-up plug of cotton wool soaked in oil of cloves to hold against the affected tooth.

Hold hot-water bottle wrapped in towel against cheek

2 Get dental help

● Advise the casualty to see his dentist as soon as possible.

Earache

This common condition is caused by inflammation inside the ear, which is often a result of an infection linked to a cold, tonsillitis, or flu, especially in children. The casualty's hearing may also be impaired, but this is usually temporary.

Your aims	You will need
▶ Relieve pain	▶ Hot-water bottle
▶ Get medical help	▶ Towel

1 Relieve pain

● An adult may take two paracetamol tablets and a child may be given the recommended dose of paracetamol syrup.
● Get the casualty to hold a hot-water bottle wrapped in a towel against his ear.

Hold hot-water bottle wrapped in towel against ear

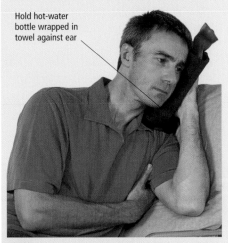

2 Get medical help

● Advise the casualty to see his doctor if the earache persists.

IMPORTANT
▶ If there is any discharge from the ear, a fever, or marked hearing loss,
✚ GET MEDICAL HELP

Headache

A headache is usually caused by tiredness and tension, but it can accompany a feverish illness, such as flu, or be part of a migraine attack (right). A headache can also be an indication of something more serious, such as a stroke (p.96) or meningitis (p.137).

Your aim	You will need
▶ Relieve pain	▶ Cold compress

1 Make casualty comfortable

● Help the casualty to sit or lie down in a quiet place.

2 Apply cold compress

● Place a cold compress (p.25) on the casualty's head.
● An adult may take two paracetamol tablets and a child may be given the recommended dose of paracetamol syrup.

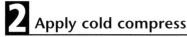
Soothe head with cold compress

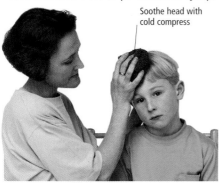

IMPORTANT
✚ CALL AN AMBULANCE
If the pain:
▶ Develops suddenly
▶ Is severe and incapacitating
▶ Is recurrent or persistent
▶ Is accompanied by a stiff neck
▶ Follows a head injury
▶ Is accompanied by a dazed feeling.

Migraine

A migraine is usually an intense, throbbing headache on one side of the head. Before an attack the casualty's vision may be disturbed. During an attack, the casualty may have nausea and vomiting and find it hard to tolerate bright light. Attacks may be triggered by a number of causes, including certain foods, such as cheese or chocolate, an allergy, or tiredness.

Your aim
▶ Relieve pain

1 Relieve pain

● If the casualty has her own medication, encourage her to take it.
● If an adult does not have her own medication, she may take two paracetamol tablets; a child may be given the recommended dose of paracetamol syrup.

2 Advise casualty to sleep

● Get the casualty to lie down in a cool, dark room and sleep for a few hours.

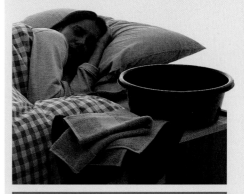

IMPORTANT
Get medical help if:
▶ It is the casualty's first migraine attack
▶ Vomiting is severe
▶ Casualty is concerned.

Sore throat

A sore throat may be the first sign of a cough or cold and will usually pass in a couple of days. It may also be caused by tonsillitis – a more serious condition – in which the tonsils at the back of the throat become infected with bacteria or viruses. The tonsils appear red and swollen, and ulcers or white spots of pus may also be visible. Swallowing may be difficult.

Your aims	You will need
▶ Relieve pain ▶ Get medical help if necessary	▶ Cool drinks

1 Give water

● Give the casualty plenty of cool drinks, particularly water, which will ease the pain and stop the throat becoming dry.
● An adult may take two paracetamol tablets and a child may be given the recommended dose of paracetamol syrup.

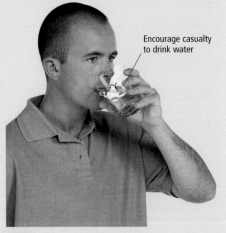

Encourage casualty to drink water

2 Get medical help

● If the pain is severe and you suspect the casualty has tonsillitis, advise him to see a doctor as soon as possible.

Fever

A fever is a body temperature that stays above the normal level of 37°C (98.6°F). It is usually a sign of an infection, either a local infection such as an abscess or a general infection such as chickenpox.

Your aims	You will need
▶ Bring down temperature ▶ Get medical help if necessary	▶ Cool, damp flannel ▶ Cool drinks

1 Bring down temperature

● Keep the casualty comfortable and cool, preferably in bed.
● Gently wipe her forehead with a cool, damp flannel.
● Give plenty of cool, bland drinks.
● An adult may take two paracetamol tablets and a child may be given the recommended dose of paracetamol syrup.

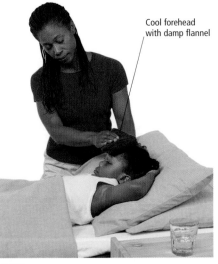

Cool forehead with damp flannel

2 Get medical help

● If the fever lasts for longer than 24 hours, the casualty should see a doctor.

Meningitis

This serious illness, which can affect anyone regardless of age, needs prompt medical treatment. It is caused by a viral or bacterial inflammation of the coverings of the brain. There are many signs and symptoms – the most common are listed below – but they are not usually all present at the same time. Without immediate treatment, permanent disability such as deafness or brain damage may result; the illness can be fatal.

Your aims	You will need
▶ Get casualty to hospital urgently ▶ Reassure casualty	▶ Cool, damp flannel

1 Call an ambulance

● If you suspect meningitis, phone for an ambulance immediately.

2 Treat the fever and reassure casualty

● Treat the fever (see opposite).
● Stay with the casualty while you wait for the ambulance.
● Keep him cool, quiet, and comfortable.

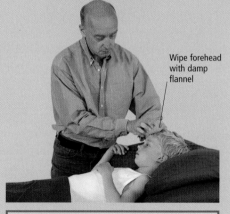

Wipe forehead with damp flannel

IMPORTANT
▶ When calling the ambulance, describe the symptoms and say that you suspect meningitis.
▶ Be prepared to insist on medical attention.
▶ If the casualty is obviously unwell and his condition worsens, even though he has already been seen by a doctor, seek urgent medical attention again.

SIGNS AND SYMPTOMS

Illness starts with:
▶ Flu-like illness
▶ High temperature
▶ Cold hands and feet, and limb pain
▶ Mottled skin

As infection develops:
▶ Headache
▶ Stiff neck (casualty cannot touch chest with chin)
▶ Vomiting
▶ Sensitivity to bright light
▶ Increasing drowsiness
▶ Distinctive rash (see Identifying the rash below).

WARNING
▶ Do not wait for all the above signs and symptoms to be present before seeking medical help.

Identifying the rash

A meningitis rash is distinctive and has the following features:
● It does not fade when pressed.
● Small red or purple pinprick spots spread to look like fresh bruising.
● It may appear late in the course of the illness or it may not come at all.
● It is not so easy to see on dark skin.

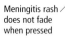

Meningitis rash does not fade when pressed

Abdominal pain

Pain in the abdomen usually indicates a relatively minor ailment such as food poisoning, but occasionally it may be a sign of a more serious condition such as appendicitis or a bowel obstruction.

Your aims	You will need
▶ Relieve pain	▶ Hot-water bottle
▶ Reassure casualty	▶ Towel
▶ Get medical help if necessary	

1 Make casualty comfortable

● Make the casualty as comfortable as you can.
● Reassure her.
● Give her a hot-water bottle wrapped in a towel to hold against the abdomen.

Soothe pain with hot-water bottle wrapped in towel

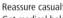

2 Get medical help

● See a doctor if the pain is severe, if the pain is accompanied by a fever and vomiting, or if you are concerned by the casualty's condition.

Vomiting and diarrhoea

These problems, which can occur together or separately, are usually the result of an irritated or infected digestive system. They may lead to dehydration, particularly if they happen at the same time, especially in infants and elderly people.

Your aims	You will need
▶ Reassure casualty	▶ Bowl
▶ Restore body fluids	▶ Warm, damp cloth
▶ Get medical help if necessary	▶ Water

1 Make casualty comfortable

● Reassure casualty.
● Give her a bowl for vomit and a warm, damp cloth for wiping her face.

2 Give drinks

● When the vomiting subsides, give the casualty plenty of clear fluids, such as water or non-fizzy drinks in frequent small sips, to restore lost body fluids.

3 Get medical help

● See a doctor if the vomiting or diarrhoea does not stop or if you are concerned by the casualty's condition.

Test yourself

Now that you have read and studied the chapter on first-aid treatments for medical problems and emergencies, see if you can answer the questions below. Check your answers against the correct ones on page 144.

1 What causes a heart attack?

....
....
....
....

2 What is the main risk associated with a heart attack?

....
....
....
....

3 Which of the following signs and symptoms indicate a heart attack?
- **a** Blueness around lips .... □
- **b** Nosebleed .... □
- **c** Breathlessness.................................... □
- **d** Blisters on the skin............................ □
- **e** Crushing pain in chest...................... □
- **f** Dizziness.. □

4 What are the priorities when treating a person known to have diabetes who is unwell but conscious?

....
....
....

5 What are the dangers to a casualty of a severe allergic reaction?

....
....
....
....

6 What might a casualty with a known severe allergy carry with him at all times?

....
....
....

7 In which of the following circumstances would you call an ambulance for a casualty who is having an asthma attack?
- **a** If the attack is severe and the casualty has trouble speaking .... □
- **b** If it is the casualty's first attack of asthma...................... □
- **c** If the casualty's breathing has not improved 5 minutes after using his inhaler................................ □
- **d** If the casualty's breathing improves quickly after using his inhaler............. □
- **e** If the casualty is becoming exhausted .... □

8 What is it most important to do when treating a high temperature (fever) and how would you do it?

....
....
....
....
....

9 If a casualty has a fever, what other signs and symptoms indicate that he or she might have meningitis?

....
....
....
....

10 Name three problems that can be helped by holding a hot-water bottle against the affected part of the body?

1 ....
2 ....
3 ....

Index

A

abdomen
  examining 19
  pain 138
abdominal thrusts
  choking
    adult 53
    child 54
agonal breathing 35
airway, opening 35
  adult 37
  child 46
  infant 50
alcohol poisoning 118
allergy 128
amputation 65
anaphylactic shock 129
angina 126
animal bites 121
ankle
  bandaging 26
  sprained 105, 112
arm
  bandaging 26
  examining 19
  fracture 108
  slings 28–9
arteries 60
assessing casualties 16–21
asthma 130

B

back
  pain 19
  spinal injury 39, 110–11
back blows
  choking
    adult 53
    child 54
    infant 55
bandages 22, 24
  roller bandages 26
  triangular bandages 27

bee stings 119
bites
  animal 121
  snake 120
"black eye" 63
bleeding 57–74
  internal bleeding 61
  nosebleed 67
  severe bleeding 58–9
  see also wounds
blisters 63
blood circulation see circulation
blood clots 60
blood vessels 60
bones, broken 101–14
brain 92
  compression 95
  concussion 94
  epilepsy 98
  fainting 97
  meningitis 137
  stroke 96
breathing 34
  asthma 130
  breathing rate 21
  checking
    adult 37
    child 46
    infant 50
  croup 131
  opening airway 35
    adult 37
    child 46
    infant 50
  rescue breathing
    adult 40–1
    child 48
    infant 51
bruising 63
burns 75–83
  chemical burns 81
  electrical burns 82
  face and head 80
  minor burns and scalds 79
  severe burns 76–7
  sunburn 83
  types of 78

C

capillaries 60
cardiac arrest 44, 124
cardiopulmonary resuscitation (CPR)
  adult 40–3
  child 49
  infant 52
casualties
  assessing 16–21
  dealing with an incident 8–9
  moving 14
  multiple casualties 14
cheekbone
  fracture 106
chemical burns 81
chest
  examining 19
chest compressions 35
  adult 40–1
  child 49
  infant 52
chest thrusts, choking
  infant 55
choking
  adult 53
  child 54
  infant 55
circulation 34,
  checking pulse 20
  resuscitation 35
clothing on fire 12
cold
  frostbite 87
  hypothermia 86–7
cold compresses 25, 63
collarbone fracture 107
compression, brain 95
concussion 94
consciousness 89–100
  AVPU code 20
  checking responses
    adult 37
    child 46
    infant 50
  see also unconsciousness

corrosive poisons 117
CPR *see* cardiopulmonary resuscitation
cramp 113
cross-infection 13
croup 131
crush injury 64
cuts and grazes 62

D

danger, assessing 10–12
defibrillators 44–5
  paediatric, 45
dehydration 84
diabetic emergency 127
diarrhoea 138
dislocated joints 104, 105
dressings 23, 24–5
drug poisoning 118

E

ear
  earache 134
  foreign object in 133
  wound 67
electrical injuries 11
  burns 82
elevation slings 29
embedded object in wound 70–1
emergency services 15
environmental injuries 75–88
epiglottitis 131
epilepsy 98
eye
  "black eye" 63
  chemical burns 81
  foreign object in 132
  wound 66

F

face
  burns 80
  fracture 106
face shield 23, 40
fainting 97
fever 136

finger *see* hand
fire 12
first-aid kit 22–3
fish-hook injury 73
foot
  bandaging 26
  cramp 113
  examining 19
foreign object
  in ear 133
  embedded object 70–1
  in eye 132
  fish-hook injury 73
  in nose 133
  splinters 72
fractures 101–14
  arm 108
  cheekbone 106
  collarbone 107
  hand 108
  jaw 106
  leg 111
  nose 106
  pelvis 109
  rib 109
  spinal injury 110–11
frostbite 87

G

gloves 13
grazes 62

H

hand
  bandaging 26, 27
  cramp 113
  examining 19
  fracture 108
  palm wound 69
  washing 13
head
  burns 80
  examining 18
  injuries 93–5
  jaw injury 106
  scalp wound 66
headache 135
heart 34
  angina 126

cardiopulmonary resuscitation
  adult 40–3
  child 48–9
  infant 51–2
defibrillators 44–5
heart attack 44, 124–5
heat exhaustion 84
heatstroke 85
hepatitis 13
high-voltage electricity 11
HIV (human immunodeficiency virus) 13
hygiene
  cross-infection 13
hyperglycaemia 127
hypoglycaemia 127
hypothermia 86–7

I

ice packs 25
immunisation, tetanus 62
incidents
  assessing casualties 16–21
  assessing dangers 10–12
  dealing with 8–9
  managing 14–15
infection, avoiding 13
insect
  in ear 133
  stings 119
insulin 127
internal bleeding 61

J

jaw injury 106
jellyfish stings 121
joint injuries 104, 105, 112

K

knee injury 113
knot, reef 22

L

leg
  bandaging 26
  cramp 113

Leg *continued*
  examining 19
  fracture 111
  knee injury 113
  sprained ankle 105, 112
life-saving techniques 31–56
ligaments, sprained 104,
  105, 112
lungs 34

M

marine injuries 121
meningitis 137
migraine 135
mouth
  burns 80
  corrosive poisons 117
  insect sting 119
  knocked-out tooth 68
  toothache 134
  wound 68
moving casualties 14
multiple casualties 14
muscle
  cramp 113
  injuries 104, 105

N

neck
  examining 18
nervous system 92
nose
  foreign object in 133
  fracture 106
  nosebleed 67

O

oxygen 34

P

palm wound 69
pelvis fracture 109
plasters 23, 25
poisoning 115–18
  alcohol or drug poisoning 118
  snake bites 120
pulse, checking 20

R

rash, meningitis 137
recovery position
  adult 38–9
  child 47
  infant 51
reef knot 22
rescue breathing
  adult 42–3
  child 48
  infant 51
resuscitation 31–52
  cardiopulmonary
    resuscitation
    adult 40–3
    child 48–9
    infant 51–2
  defibrillators 44–5
  rescue breathing
    adult 42–3
    child 48
    infant 51
rib
  fracture 109
roller bandages 26

S

safety
  assessing dangers
    10–12
scalds 76, 79
scalp wound 66
sea urchins 121
seizures
  child 99
shock 61
  anaphylactic 129
skin
  burns 75–83
skull
  head injuries 93–5
slings 28–9
snake bites 120
sore throat 136
spinal injury 39,
  110–11
spines
  marine injuries 121
splinters 72

sprained joints 104,
  105
  ankle 112
sterilising tweezers 72
stimulant drugs 118
stings
  insect 119
  marine injuries 121
strains 104, 105
stress, coping with 15
stroke 96
sunburn 83

T

temperature
  fever 136
  frostbite 87
  heat exhaustion 84
  heatstroke 85
  hypothermia 86–7
  thermometers 21
tendon injuries 104,
  105
tetanus immunisation 62
thermometers 21
throat
  burns 80
  insect stings 119
  sore throat 136
tonsillitis 136
tooth
  bleeding socket 68
  knocked-out 68
  toothache 134
traffic incidents 10
triangular bandages 27
tweezers, sterilising 72

U

unconsciousness
  AVPU code 20
  checking responses
    adult 37
    child 46
    infant 50
  collapsed person 90–1
  dealing with 32–3
  diabetic emergency 127
  epilepsy 98

fainting 97
head injury 93, 95
recovery position
  adult 38–9
  child 47
  infant 51
seizures
  child 99
spinal injury 111
stroke 96

V

veins 60
viruses
  avoiding cross-infection 13
vital signs, monitoring 20–1
vomiting 138

W

wasp stings 119
waste disposal 13
water
  dehydration 84
  rescuing casualties 10
weever fish 121
wounds 57–74
  amputation 65
  animal bites 121
  avoiding cross-infection 13
  cuts and grazes 62
  ear 67
  embedded object 70–1
  eye 66
  fish-hook injury 73
  mouth 68
  palm 69
  scalp 66
  splinters 72

Acknowledgments

The author would like to thank Dr J Gordon Paterson FFPHM FRCPE DRCOG DCM; Joe Mulligan, Head of First Aid Services, British Red Cross; Ken Sharpe, Head of First Aid Technical Support Unit, British Red Cross; Katrina Thornton, Head of Purchasing and Supply, British Red Cross; and Charlotte Hall, Head of First Aid Marketing and Service Support Unit, British Red Cross

Cooling Brown would like to thank Evelynne Stoikou and Sally Tynan for the models' make-up, Patsy North for proofreading, and Hilary Bird for compiling the index

Previous edition Jolyon Goddard, Sara Kimmins, and Julian Dams at Dorling Kindersley; Amanda Lebentz, Helen Ridge, and Elly King at Cooling Brown

Models Francesca Agati, Christine Appella, Angela Cameron, Madelane Cameron, Scott Davis, Emma Forge, Jessica Forge, Mark Ireland, Alastair King, Natalie King, Olivia King, Crispin Lord, Philip Lord, Eric Lowes, Kincaid Malik-White, Tony Mayne, Camilla Moore, Juliette Norsworthy, Sagaren Pillay, Anna Pizzi, Eleanor Ridge, Sheila Tait, Suki Tan, Peter Taylor, Jeremy Wallis, Tim Webster

Illustrator Patrick Mulrey

Photographers Trish Gant, Steve Gorton, Dave King, Gary Ombler, Matthew Ward
All other images © Dorling Kindersley.
For further information see: **www.dkimages.com**

The British Red Cross helps people in crisis whoever and wherever they are. We are part of a global network of volunteers responding to natural disasters, conflicts, and individual emergencies. The Red Cross is also the world's leading First Aid training provider, helping people prepare for, and respond to, accidents and emergencies. The red cross emblem is a symbol of protection during armed conflict and its use is restricted by law.

Test yourself: answers

Chapter 1 First-aid principles, page 30
1 Make sure that you are not in danger. 2 Call the emergency services and do not approach the scene of the incident. 3 The quietest ones because they may be unconscious. 4 Disposable gloves. 5 A specially designed yellow box used for the disposal of hypodermic needles and other sharp objects. 6 Dial 999 and ask for the relevant service (fire, ambulance, or police). 7 A = Alert; V = Voice; P = Pain; U = Unresponsive. 8 At the wrist (radial pulse), at the neck (carotid pulse), or in babies on the inside of the upper arm (brachial pulse). 9 a; c; d; and f. A blanket (b) and scissors (e) are useful additions but not basic requirements. 10 Because it will not slip and is easy to undo. Also, since it lies flat against the body it is more comfortable for the casualty. 11 The ice will burn the skin. 12 Press the skin of the finger or toe until it turns pale and then watch for colour to return. 13 Arm sling: to support an injured upper arm, forearm, or wrist and to immobilise an arm if there is a chest injury. Elevation sling: to support the arm in a raised position when a hand or forearm is injured and bleeding needs to be controlled; to support a broken hand; to reduce swelling in an injured arm; to support an arm in the event of a broken collarbone or rib.

Chapter 2 Life-saving techniques, page 56
1 Airway, breathing, and circulation. 2 Heart. 3 Open the airway; check breathing; put the casualty in the recovery position; then call an ambulance. 4 One second 5 When giving rescue breaths, a face shield will prevent cross-infection. 6 Cardiopulmonary resuscitation, which is a combination of rescue breathing and chest compressions. 7 Centre of the chest. 8 For an adult, give 30 compressions then two rescue breaths. For a child or an infant, give five rescue breaths first, then 30 chest compressions followed by two rescue breaths. For a casualty of any age, chest compressions should be given at a rate of 100 per minute. 9 A machine that restarts a heart that has an abnormal heart rhythm (known as ventricular fibrillation). 10 a; c; d; and f. 11 Abdominal thrusts.

Chapter 3 Wounds and bleeding, page 74
1 c; a; and then e. 2 Cover with a second dressing. If blood seeps through the second dressing, remove both and apply a new one. 3 Arteries; capillaries; veins. 4 Shock. 5 Rinse the wound, clean around it with a fresh swab or wipe, pick out any loose foreign matter, and cover with a plaster or sterile wound dressing. To prevent cross-infection, you should also wear disposable gloves when treating the casualty. 6 Level of response; pulse; and breathing. 7 To reduce blood flow to the bruise, thereby reducing swelling and pain. 8 Lean forwards; pinch the soft part of the nose. 9 a or b. 10 A skull fracture. 11 Pinch the edges of the wound together around the embedded object.

Chapter 4 Environmental injuries, page 88
1 Cool the burn, prevent infection, treat any signs of shock, and get medical help. 2 Superficial burn; partial-thickness burn; full-thickness burn. 3 Fluid loss leading to shock. 4 Do not apply creams, sprays, ointments, or adhesive tape to the burn; do not touch the burnt area; do not remove any clothing sticking to the burn. 5 Clean plastic bag, clean tea towel, clean sheet, or kitchen film. 6 Damaged skin and/or soot around the mouth. 7 Cool for at least 10 minutes. If you cool a burn for too long, there is a risk of hypothermia. 8 At least 20 minutes to wash off all the chemical. 9 Break the casualty's contact with the electricity. 10 Dehydration. 11 Signs and symptoms include loss of consciousness; very cold, pale skin; shivering; clumsiness; irritability; slurred speech; slow breathing; weak pulse; and lethargy. 12 To warm the affected part slowly and to get the casualty to hospital.

Chapter 5 Disorders affecting consciousness, page 100
1 They can affect the casualty's level of consciousness. 2 Bruising and/or bleeding of the scalp; concussion; compression; fracture to the skull; injury to the spine. 3 The casualty's level of response deteriorates after a head injury. 4 The casualty is dazed and confused, probably for a few minutes, before making a full recovery. 5 Open the casualty's airway, check his breathing, and be ready to begin resuscitation if necessary. 6 b and c. 7 A brief loss of consciousness due to the reduced flow of blood to the brain. 8 c. 9 Protect the child from injury; cool him; call an ambulance. 10 Level of response; pulse; and breathing.

Chapter 6 Bone, joint, and muscle injuries, page 114
1 a and d. 2 An injury in which a bone is broken along with a break in the skin, sometimes with the bone protruding. 3 Infection. 4 The casualty may later need a general anaesthetic. 5 A sprain is a torn ligament (a fibrous band that holds bones together at a joint) and a strain is an overstretched muscle or tendon (a fibrous band that attaches a muscle to a bone). 6 As a result of an indirect force, for example from falling onto an outstretched hand. 7 Pain and tenderness; reluctance to move injured arm; deformity, swelling, and bruising. 8 Internal bleeding and shock. 9 Keep the affected part still to prevent broken bone ends causing further damage to blood vessels, tissues, or internal organs. 10 Rest; Ice; Compress; Elevate. 11 For 10 minutes and reassess the injury. Reapply at 10-minute intervals for up to 30 minutes if necessary. 12 Straighten the casualty's knee and pull the foot up towards the shin as far as possible, and then gently massage the calf muscles.

Chapter 7 Poisoning, bites, and stings, page 122
1 Identify poison, get casualty to hospital urgently, and monitor casualty regularly until help arrives. 2 Use a face shield or the mouth-to-nose method. 3 All of them. 4 Hypothermia may develop. 5 Lower the casualty's body temperature by getting him to rest in a cool place. 6 Scrape it away with your fingernail or a rigid piece of plastic, such as a credit card. 7 Because they may squeeze more venom into the casualty. 8 The swelling it causes can block the casualty's airway. 9 Keep the casualty still; keep her heart above the level of the bite; bandage above the bite. 10 Tetanus and rabies. 11 Get the casualty to sit or lie down and cover the sting with an ice pack. 12 Pour lots of vinegar or sea water over the wound, lightly cover the sting with a roller bandage, and call an ambulance.

Chapter 8 Medical problems and emergencies, page 139
1 A blockage in an artery carrying blood to part of the heart muscle. 2 That the casualty will lose consciousness because the heart will stop beating (cardiac arrest). 3 a; c; e; and f. 4 Give the casualty a sugary drink or something sweet to eat. 5 Breathing difficulties and loss of consciousness. 6 Auto-injector containing epinephrine (adrenaline). 7 a; b; c; and e. 8 Cool the casualty by wiping the forehead with a cool, damp cloth and giving plenty of cool drinks. In addition, an adult may take two paracetamol tablets and a child the recommended dose of paracetamol syrup. 9 As illness starts: flu-like illness, high temperature, cold hands and feet, with limb pain, mottled skin. As infection develops: headache, stiff neck, vomiting, sensitivity to bright light, increasing drowsiness, distinctive rash. 10 Toothache; earache; abdominal pain.